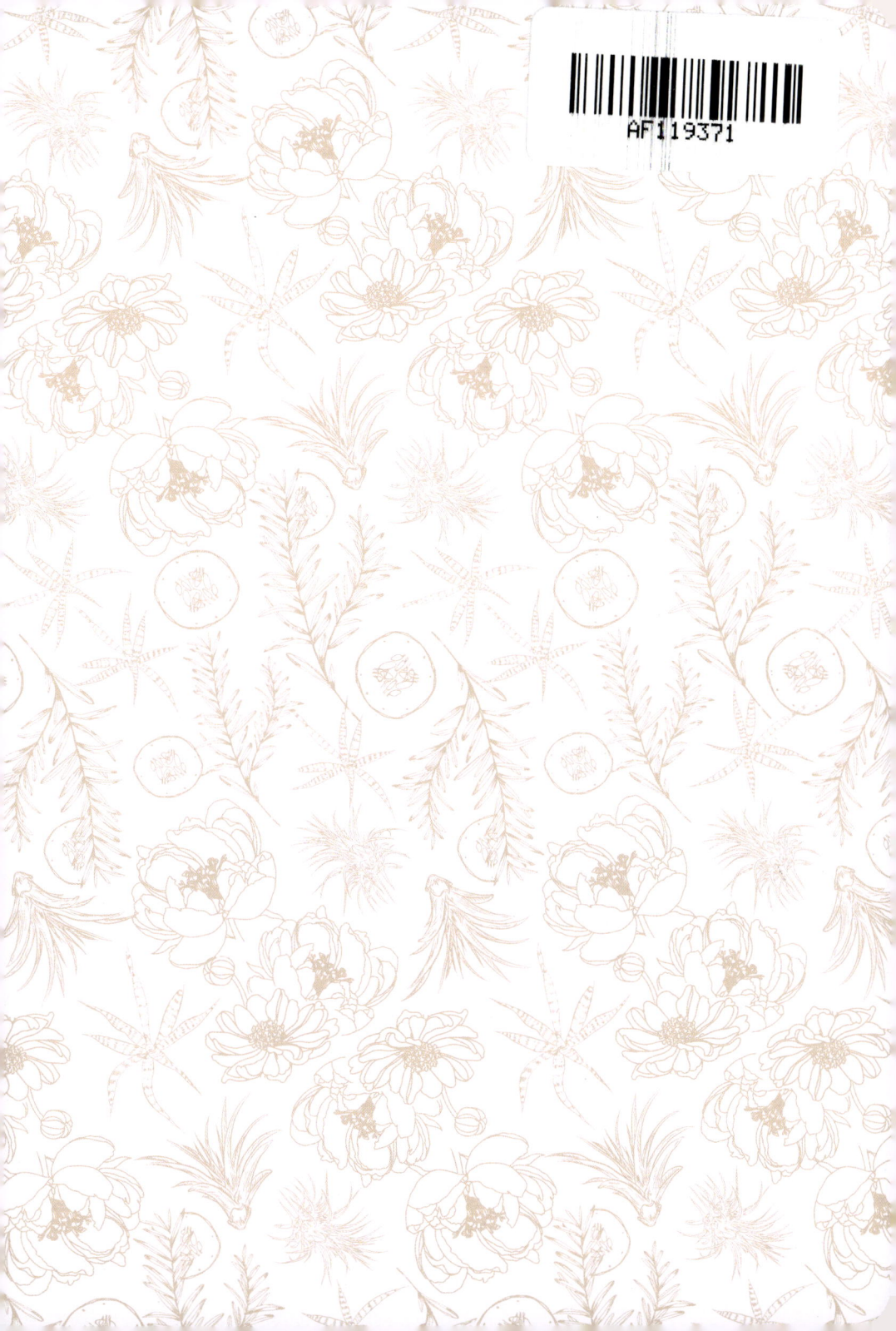

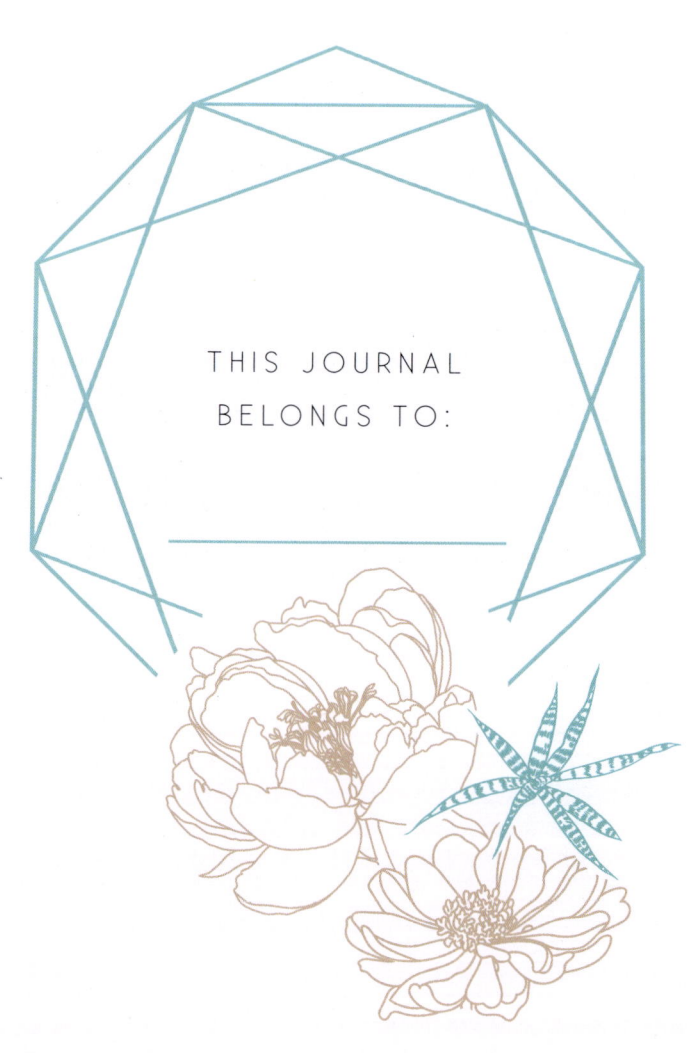

THIS JOURNAL BELONGS TO:

SELF-CARE

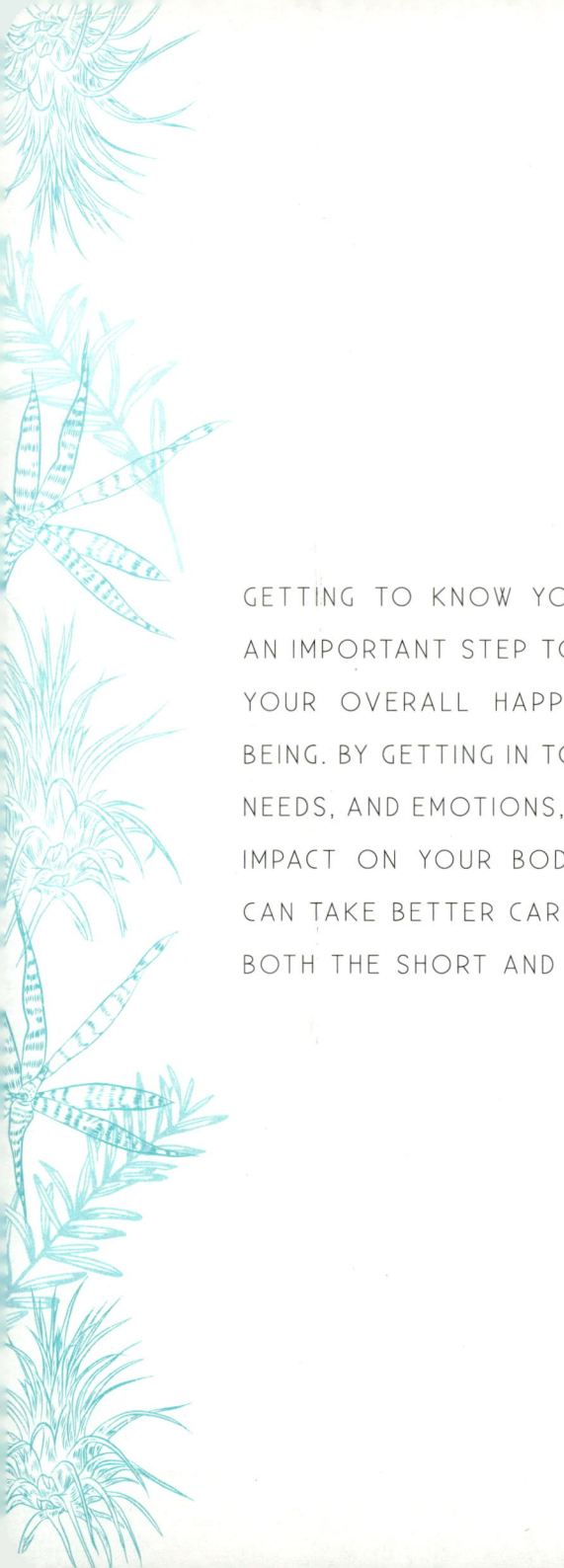

GETTING TO KNOW YOUR INNER SELF IS AN IMPORTANT STEP TOWARD INCREASING YOUR OVERALL HAPPINESS AND WELL-BEING. BY GETTING IN TOUCH WITH HABITS, NEEDS, AND EMOTIONS, AS WELL AS THEIR IMPACT ON YOUR BODY AND MIND, YOU CAN TAKE BETTER CARE OF YOURSELF IN BOTH THE SHORT AND LONG TERM.

Your physical and mental health is shaped by diet, sleep, exercise, and other activities. This journal provides a space for daily observations and reflections on how you spend your time and how you care for yourself. It will help you track the impact of your habits and lifestyle on how you feel physically and mentally in order to find out how to be the healthiest and happiest you can be.

The way you use this journal will depend on your individual lifestyle. You can carry it with you and make notes in real time or reflect back on your day before bed. Savor the chance to get to know yourself better, and cherish the ways you can care for yourself.

RECORD

DATE ___/___/___

AN INTENTION FOR THE DAY:

SLEPT: FROM ___:___ TO ___:___   TOTAL HOURS:___

☐ GOOD DREAMS   ☐ BAD DREAMS   ☐ NO DREAMS

NOTES:

WHAT I ATE FOR:

BREAKFAST:

LUNCH:

DINNER:

SNACKS:

NUMBER OF CUPS OF WATER I DRANK: ___

EXERCISE: FROM ___:___ TO ___:___
TOTAL MINUTES: ___
TYPE:

OTHER ACTIVITIES:

- ☐ JOURNALING
- ☐ SOCIAL TIME
- ☐ MEDITATION
- ☐ GRATITUDE
- ☐ TIME OUTSIDE
- ☐ CREATIVE WORK
- ☐ SPIRITUAL PRACTICE
- ☐ SPA TIME
- ☐ THERAPY
- ☐ ALONE TIME
- ☐ BEING SILLY
- ☐ LEARNING SOMETHING NEW
- ☐ LISTENING TO MUSIC
- ☐ COOKING
- ☐ CLEANING
- ☐ _____

REFLECT

PHYSICALLY, I FEEL:

- [ ] ENERGIZED
- [ ] WELL-RESTED
- [ ] STRONG
- [ ] LIMBER
- [ ] RELAXED
- [ ] _____

- [ ] SLUGGISH
- [ ] TIRED
- [ ] WEAK
- [ ] SORE
- [ ] STRESSED
- [ ] _____

THINGS THAT WERE FUN OR RELAXING TODAY:

OTHER THOUGHTS:

THINGS THAT WERE HARD OR STRESSFUL TODAY:

KIND THINGS I DID FOR MYSELF:

TIME:	AS I WOKE UP			AS I WENT TO SLEEP
MOOD:				
NOTES:				

RECORD

DATE ___/___/___

AN INTENTION FOR THE DAY:

SLEPT: FROM ___:___ TO ___:___   TOTAL HOURS:___
☐ GOOD DREAMS   ☐ BAD DREAMS   ☐ NO DREAMS
NOTES:

WHAT I ATE FOR:

BREAKFAST:	LUNCH:
DINNER:	SNACKS:

NUMBER OF CUPS OF WATER I DRANK: ___

EXERCISE: FROM ___:___ TO ___:___
TOTAL MINUTES: ___
TYPE:

OTHER ACTIVITIES:

☐ JOURNALING   ☐ SPIRITUAL   ☐ LEARNING
☐ SOCIAL TIME   PRACTICE   SOMETHING NEW
☐ MEDITATION   ☐ SPA TIME   ☐ LISTENING TO MUSIC
☐ GRATITUDE   ☐ THERAPY   ☐ COOKING
☐ TIME OUTSIDE   ☐ ALONE TIME   ☐ CLEANING
☐ CREATIVE WORK   ☐ BEING SILLY   ☐ _____

REFLECT

PHYSICALLY, I FEEL:

- [ ] ENERGIZED
- [ ] WELL-RESTED
- [ ] STRONG
- [ ] LIMBER
- [ ] RELAXED
- [ ] _____

- [ ] SLUGGISH
- [ ] TIRED
- [ ] WEAK
- [ ] SORE
- [ ] STRESSED
- [ ] _____

THINGS THAT WERE FUN OR RELAXING TODAY:
_____
_____
_____

THINGS THAT WERE HARD OR STRESSFUL TODAY:
_____
_____
_____

KIND THINGS I DID FOR MYSELF:
_____
_____
_____

OTHER THOUGHTS:
_____
_____
_____
_____
_____
_____

TIME:	AS I WOKE UP			AS I WENT TO SLEEP
MOOD:				
NOTES:				

RECORD

DATE ___/___/___

AN INTENTION FOR THE DAY:

SLEPT: FROM ___:___ TO ___:___   TOTAL HOURS:___

☐ GOOD DREAMS   ☐ BAD DREAMS   ☐ NO DREAMS

NOTES:

WHAT I ATE FOR:

BREAKFAST:

LUNCH:

DINNER:

SNACKS:

NUMBER OF CUPS OF WATER I DRANK: ___

EXERCISE: FROM ___:___ TO ___:___
TOTAL MINUTES: ___
TYPE:

OTHER ACTIVITIES:

☐ JOURNALING
☐ SOCIAL TIME
☐ MEDITATION
☐ GRATITUDE
☐ TIME OUTSIDE
☐ CREATIVE WORK

☐ SPIRITUAL PRACTICE
☐ SPA TIME
☐ THERAPY
☐ ALONE TIME
☐ BEING SILLY

☐ LEARNING SOMETHING NEW
☐ LISTENING TO MUSIC
☐ COOKING
☐ CLEANING
☐ _____

REFLECT

PHYSICALLY, I FEEL:

- ☐ ENERGIZED
- ☐ WELL-RESTED
- ☐ STRONG
- ☐ LIMBER
- ☐ RELAXED
- ☐ _____

- ☐ SLUGGISH
- ☐ TIRED
- ☐ WEAK
- ☐ SORE
- ☐ STRESSED
- ☐ _____

THINGS THAT WERE FUN OR RELAXING TODAY:
_____
_____
_____

THINGS THAT WERE HARD OR STRESSFUL TODAY:
_____
_____
_____

KIND THINGS I DID FOR MYSELF:
_____
_____
_____

OTHER THOUGHTS:
_____
_____
_____
_____
_____
_____
_____

TIME:	AS I WOKE UP			AS I WENT TO SLEEP
MOOD:				
NOTES:				

RECORD

DATE ___/___/___

AN INTENTION FOR THE DAY:

SLEPT: FROM ___:___ TO ___:___ TOTAL HOURS:___

☐ GOOD DREAMS ☐ BAD DREAMS ☐ NO DREAMS

NOTES: _____

WHAT I ATE FOR:

BREAKFAST:

LUNCH:

DINNER:

SNACKS:

NUMBER OF CUPS OF WATER I DRANK: ___

EXERCISE: FROM ___:___ TO ___:___
TOTAL MINUTES: ___
TYPE:

OTHER ACTIVITIES:

☐ JOURNALING
☐ SOCIAL TIME
☐ MEDITATION
☐ GRATITUDE
☐ TIME OUTSIDE
☐ CREATIVE WORK

☐ SPIRITUAL PRACTICE
☐ SPA TIME
☐ THERAPY
☐ ALONE TIME
☐ BEING SILLY

☐ LEARNING SOMETHING NEW
☐ LISTENING TO MUSIC
☐ COOKING
☐ CLEANING
☐ _____

REFLECT

PHYSICALLY, I FEEL:

- [ ] ENERGIZED
- [ ] WELL-RESTED
- [ ] STRONG
- [ ] LIMBER
- [ ] RELAXED
- [ ] _____

- [ ] SLUGGISH
- [ ] TIRED
- [ ] WEAK
- [ ] SORE
- [ ] STRESSED
- [ ] _____

THINGS THAT WERE FUN OR RELAXING TODAY:
_____
_____
_____

THINGS THAT WERE HARD OR STRESSFUL TODAY:
_____
_____
_____

KIND THINGS I DID FOR MYSELF:
_____
_____
_____

OTHER THOUGHTS:
_____
_____
_____
_____
_____
_____
_____

TIME:	AS I WOKE UP			AS I WENT TO SLEEP
MOOD:				
NOTES:				

RECORD

DATE ___/___/___

AN INTENTION FOR THE DAY:

SLEPT: FROM ___:___ TO ___:___   TOTAL HOURS:___
☐ GOOD DREAMS   ☐ BAD DREAMS   ☐ NO DREAMS
NOTES:

WHAT I ATE FOR:

BREAKFAST:

LUNCH:

DINNER:

SNACKS:

NUMBER OF CUPS OF WATER I DRANK:___

EXERCISE: FROM ___:___ TO ___:___
TOTAL MINUTES:___
TYPE:

OTHER ACTIVITIES:

☐ JOURNALING
☐ SOCIAL TIME
☐ MEDITATION
☐ GRATITUDE
☐ TIME OUTSIDE
☐ CREATIVE WORK

☐ SPIRITUAL PRACTICE
☐ SPA TIME
☐ THERAPY
☐ ALONE TIME
☐ BEING SILLY

☐ LEARNING SOMETHING NEW
☐ LISTENING TO MUSIC
☐ COOKING
☐ CLEANING
☐ _____

REFLECT

PHYSICALLY, I FEEL:

- [ ] ENERGIZED
- [ ] WELL-RESTED
- [ ] STRONG
- [ ] LIMBER
- [ ] RELAXED
- [ ] _____

- [ ] SLUGGISH
- [ ] TIRED
- [ ] WEAK
- [ ] SORE
- [ ] STRESSED
- [ ] _____

THINGS THAT WERE FUN OR RELAXING TODAY:
_____
_____
_____

OTHER THOUGHTS:
_____
_____
_____

THINGS THAT WERE HARD OR STRESSFUL TODAY:
_____
_____
_____

_____
_____
_____

KIND THINGS I DID FOR MYSELF:
_____
_____
_____

TIME:	AS I WOKE UP			AS I WENT TO SLEEP
MOOD:				
NOTES:				

RECORD

DATE ___/___/___

AN INTENTION FOR THE DAY:

SLEPT: FROM ___:___ TO ___:___   TOTAL HOURS: ___

☐ GOOD DREAMS   ☐ BAD DREAMS   ☐ NO DREAMS

NOTES:

WHAT I ATE FOR:

BREAKFAST:

LUNCH:

DINNER:

SNACKS:

NUMBER OF CUPS OF WATER I DRANK: ___

EXERCISE: FROM ___:___ TO ___:___
TOTAL MINUTES: ___
TYPE:

OTHER ACTIVITIES:

☐ JOURNALING
☐ SOCIAL TIME
☐ MEDITATION
☐ GRATITUDE
☐ TIME OUTSIDE
☐ CREATIVE WORK

☐ SPIRITUAL PRACTICE
☐ SPA TIME
☐ THERAPY
☐ ALONE TIME
☐ BEING SILLY

☐ LEARNING SOMETHING NEW
☐ LISTENING TO MUSIC
☐ COOKING
☐ CLEANING
☐ _____

REFLECT

PHYSICALLY, I FEEL:

- [ ] ENERGIZED
- [ ] WELL-RESTED
- [ ] STRONG
- [ ] LIMBER
- [ ] RELAXED
- [ ] _____

- [ ] SLUGGISH
- [ ] TIRED
- [ ] WEAK
- [ ] SORE
- [ ] STRESSED
- [ ] _____

THINGS THAT WERE FUN OR RELAXING TODAY:
_____
_____
_____

THINGS THAT WERE HARD OR STRESSFUL TODAY:
_____
_____
_____

KIND THINGS I DID FOR MYSELF:
_____
_____
_____

OTHER THOUGHTS:
_____
_____
_____
_____
_____
_____
_____

TIME:	AS I WOKE UP			AS I WENT TO SLEEP
MOOD:				
NOTES:				

RECORD

DATE ___/___/___

AN INTENTION FOR THE DAY:

SLEPT: FROM ___:___ TO ___:___   TOTAL HOURS:___
☐ GOOD DREAMS ☐ BAD DREAMS ☐ NO DREAMS
NOTES:

WHAT I ATE FOR:

BREAKFAST:

LUNCH:

DINNER:

SNACKS:

NUMBER OF CUPS OF WATER I DRANK: ___

EXERCISE: FROM ___:___ TO ___:___
TOTAL MINUTES: ___
TYPE:

OTHER ACTIVITIES:

☐ JOURNALING
☐ SOCIAL TIME
☐ MEDITATION
☐ GRATITUDE
☐ TIME OUTSIDE
☐ CREATIVE WORK

☐ SPIRITUAL PRACTICE
☐ SPA TIME
☐ THERAPY
☐ ALONE TIME
☐ BEING SILLY

☐ LEARNING SOMETHING NEW
☐ LISTENING TO MUSIC
☐ COOKING
☐ CLEANING
☐ _____

REFLECT

PHYSICALLY, I FEEL:

- ☐ ENERGIZED
- ☐ WELL-RESTED
- ☐ STRONG
- ☐ LIMBER
- ☐ RELAXED
- ☐ _____

- ☐ SLUGGISH
- ☐ TIRED
- ☐ WEAK
- ☐ SORE
- ☐ STRESSED
- ☐ _____

THINGS THAT WERE FUN OR RELAXING TODAY:
_____
_____
_____

OTHER THOUGHTS:
_____
_____
_____
_____
_____
_____
_____

THINGS THAT WERE HARD OR STRESSFUL TODAY:
_____
_____
_____

KIND THINGS I DID FOR MYSELF:
_____
_____
_____

TIME:	AS I WOKE UP			AS I WENT TO SLEEP
MOOD:				
NOTES:				

RECORD

DATE ___/___/___

AN INTENTION FOR THE DAY:

SLEPT: FROM ___:___ TO ___:___ TOTAL HOURS:___
☐ GOOD DREAMS ☐ BAD DREAMS ☐ NO DREAMS
NOTES:

WHAT I ATE FOR:

BREAKFAST:

LUNCH:

DINNER:

SNACKS:

NUMBER OF CUPS OF WATER I DRANK: ___

EXERCISE: FROM ___:___ TO ___:___
TOTAL MINUTES: ___
TYPE:

OTHER ACTIVITIES:

☐ JOURNALING
☐ SOCIAL TIME
☐ MEDITATION
☐ GRATITUDE
☐ TIME OUTSIDE
☐ CREATIVE WORK
☐ SPIRITUAL PRACTICE
☐ SPA TIME
☐ THERAPY
☐ ALONE TIME
☐ BEING SILLY
☐ LEARNING SOMETHING NEW
☐ LISTENING TO MUSIC
☐ COOKING
☐ CLEANING
☐ _____

REFLECT

PHYSICALLY, I FEEL:

- [ ] ENERGIZED
- [ ] WELL-RESTED
- [ ] STRONG
- [ ] LIMBER
- [ ] RELAXED
- [ ] _____

- [ ] SLUGGISH
- [ ] TIRED
- [ ] WEAK
- [ ] SORE
- [ ] STRESSED
- [ ] _____

THINGS THAT WERE FUN OR RELAXING TODAY:
_____
_____
_____

OTHER THOUGHTS:
_____
_____
_____
_____
_____
_____
_____
_____

THINGS THAT WERE HARD OR STRESSFUL TODAY:
_____
_____
_____

KIND THINGS I DID FOR MYSELF:
_____
_____
_____

TIME:	AS I WOKE UP			AS I WENT TO SLEEP
MOOD:				
NOTES:				

RECORD

DATE ___/___/___

AN INTENTION FOR THE DAY:

SLEPT: FROM ___:___ TO ___:___   TOTAL HOURS:___

☐ GOOD DREAMS   ☐ BAD DREAMS   ☐ NO DREAMS

NOTES:

WHAT I ATE FOR:

BREAKFAST:

LUNCH:

DINNER:

SNACKS:

NUMBER OF CUPS OF WATER I DRANK: ___

EXERCISE: FROM ___:___ TO ___:___

TOTAL MINUTES: ___

TYPE:

OTHER ACTIVITIES:

- ☐ JOURNALING
- ☐ SOCIAL TIME
- ☐ MEDITATION
- ☐ GRATITUDE
- ☐ TIME OUTSIDE
- ☐ CREATIVE WORK
- ☐ SPIRITUAL PRACTICE
- ☐ SPA TIME
- ☐ THERAPY
- ☐ ALONE TIME
- ☐ BEING SILLY
- ☐ LEARNING SOMETHING NEW
- ☐ LISTENING TO MUSIC
- ☐ COOKING
- ☐ CLEANING
- ☐ _____

REFLECT

PHYSICALLY, I FEEL:

- [ ] ENERGIZED
- [ ] WELL-RESTED
- [ ] STRONG
- [ ] LIMBER
- [ ] RELAXED
- [ ] _____

- [ ] SLUGGISH
- [ ] TIRED
- [ ] WEAK
- [ ] SORE
- [ ] STRESSED
- [ ] _____

THINGS THAT WERE FUN OR RELAXING TODAY:
_____
_____
_____

THINGS THAT WERE HARD OR STRESSFUL TODAY:
_____
_____
_____

KIND THINGS I DID FOR MYSELF:
_____
_____
_____

OTHER THOUGHTS:
_____
_____
_____
_____
_____
_____

TIME:	AS I WOKE UP			AS I WENT TO SLEEP
MOOD:				
NOTES:				

RECORD

DATE ___/___/___

AN INTENTION FOR THE DAY:

SLEPT: FROM ___:___ TO ___:___   TOTAL HOURS:___
☐ GOOD DREAMS   ☐ BAD DREAMS   ☐ NO DREAMS
NOTES:

WHAT I ATE FOR:

BREAKFAST:

LUNCH:

DINNER:

SNACKS:

NUMBER OF CUPS OF WATER I DRANK: ___

EXERCISE: FROM ___:___ TO ___:___
TOTAL MINUTES: ___
TYPE:

OTHER ACTIVITIES:

☐ JOURNALING
☐ SOCIAL TIME
☐ MEDITATION
☐ GRATITUDE
☐ TIME OUTSIDE
☐ CREATIVE WORK
☐ SPIRITUAL PRACTICE
☐ SPA TIME
☐ THERAPY
☐ ALONE TIME
☐ BEING SILLY
☐ LEARNING SOMETHING NEW
☐ LISTENING TO MUSIC
☐ COOKING
☐ CLEANING
☐ _____

REFLECT

PHYSICALLY, I FEEL:

- [ ] ENERGIZED
- [ ] WELL-RESTED
- [ ] STRONG
- [ ] LIMBER
- [ ] RELAXED
- [ ] _____

- [ ] SLUGGISH
- [ ] TIRED
- [ ] WEAK
- [ ] SORE
- [ ] STRESSED
- [ ] _____

THINGS THAT WERE FUN OR RELAXING TODAY:
_____
_____
_____

THINGS THAT WERE HARD OR STRESSFUL TODAY:
_____
_____
_____

KIND THINGS I DID FOR MYSELF:
_____
_____
_____

OTHER THOUGHTS:
_____
_____
_____
_____
_____
_____
_____

TIME:	AS I WOKE UP			AS I WENT TO SLEEP
MOOD:				
NOTES:				

RECORD

DATE ___/___/___

AN INTENTION FOR THE DAY:

SLEPT: FROM ___:___ TO ___:___   TOTAL HOURS:___

☐ GOOD DREAMS ☐ BAD DREAMS ☐ NO DREAMS

NOTES:

WHAT I ATE FOR:

BREAKFAST:

LUNCH:

DINNER:

SNACKS:

NUMBER OF CUPS OF WATER I DRANK: ___

EXERCISE: FROM ___:___ TO ___:___
TOTAL MINUTES: ___
TYPE:

OTHER ACTIVITIES:

☐ JOURNALING
☐ SOCIAL TIME
☐ MEDITATION
☐ GRATITUDE
☐ TIME OUTSIDE
☐ CREATIVE WORK

☐ SPIRITUAL PRACTICE
☐ SPA TIME
☐ THERAPY
☐ ALONE TIME
☐ BEING SILLY

☐ LEARNING SOMETHING NEW
☐ LISTENING TO MUSIC
☐ COOKING
☐ CLEANING
☐ _____

REFLECT

PHYSICALLY, I FEEL:

- [ ] ENERGIZED
- [ ] WELL-RESTED
- [ ] STRONG
- [ ] LIMBER
- [ ] RELAXED
- [ ] _____

- [ ] SLUGGISH
- [ ] TIRED
- [ ] WEAK
- [ ] SORE
- [ ] STRESSED
- [ ] _____

THINGS THAT WERE FUN OR RELAXING TODAY:
_____
_____
_____

THINGS THAT WERE HARD OR STRESSFUL TODAY:
_____
_____
_____

KIND THINGS I DID FOR MYSELF:
_____
_____
_____

OTHER THOUGHTS:
_____
_____
_____
_____
_____
_____
_____

TIME:	AS I WOKE UP			AS I WENT TO SLEEP
MOOD:				
NOTES:				

RECORD

DATE ___/___/___

AN INTENTION FOR THE DAY:

SLEPT: FROM ___:___ TO ___:___   TOTAL HOURS:___
☐ GOOD DREAMS   ☐ BAD DREAMS   ☐ NO DREAMS
NOTES:

WHAT I ATE FOR:

BREAKFAST:

LUNCH:

DINNER:

SNACKS:

NUMBER OF CUPS OF WATER I DRANK: ___

EXERCISE: FROM ___:___ TO ___:___
TOTAL MINUTES: ___
TYPE:

OTHER ACTIVITIES:

☐ JOURNALING
☐ SOCIAL TIME
☐ MEDITATION
☐ GRATITUDE
☐ TIME OUTSIDE
☐ CREATIVE WORK

☐ SPIRITUAL PRACTICE
☐ SPA TIME
☐ THERAPY
☐ ALONE TIME
☐ BEING SILLY

☐ LEARNING SOMETHING NEW
☐ LISTENING TO MUSIC
☐ COOKING
☐ CLEANING
☐ _____

REFLECT

PHYSICALLY, I FEEL:

- ☐ ENERGIZED
- ☐ WELL-RESTED
- ☐ STRONG
- ☐ LIMBER
- ☐ RELAXED
- ☐ _____

- ☐ SLUGGISH
- ☐ TIRED
- ☐ WEAK
- ☐ SORE
- ☐ STRESSED
- ☐ _____

THINGS THAT WERE FUN OR RELAXING TODAY:
_____
_____
_____

THINGS THAT WERE HARD OR STRESSFUL TODAY:
_____
_____
_____

KIND THINGS I DID FOR MYSELF:
_____
_____
_____

OTHER THOUGHTS:
_____
_____
_____
_____
_____
_____
_____

TIME:	AS I WOKE UP			AS I WENT TO SLEEP
MOOD:				
NOTES:				

RECORD

DATE ___/___/___

AN INTENTION FOR THE DAY:

SLEPT: FROM ___:___ TO ___:___ TOTAL HOURS:___
☐ GOOD DREAMS ☐ BAD DREAMS ☐ NO DREAMS
NOTES:

WHAT I ATE FOR:

BREAKFAST:

LUNCH:

DINNER:

SNACKS:

NUMBER OF CUPS OF WATER I DRANK: ___

EXERCISE: FROM ___:___ TO ___:___
TOTAL MINUTES: ___
TYPE:

OTHER ACTIVITIES:

☐ JOURNALING
☐ SOCIAL TIME
☐ MEDITATION
☐ GRATITUDE
☐ TIME OUTSIDE
☐ CREATIVE WORK

☐ SPIRITUAL PRACTICE
☐ SPA TIME
☐ THERAPY
☐ ALONE TIME
☐ BEING SILLY

☐ LEARNING SOMETHING NEW
☐ LISTENING TO MUSIC
☐ COOKING
☐ CLEANING
☐ _____

REFLECT

PHYSICALLY, I FEEL:

- [ ] ENERGIZED
- [ ] WELL-RESTED
- [ ] STRONG
- [ ] LIMBER
- [ ] RELAXED
- [ ] _____

- [ ] SLUGGISH
- [ ] TIRED
- [ ] WEAK
- [ ] SORE
- [ ] STRESSED
- [ ] _____

THINGS THAT WERE FUN OR RELAXING TODAY:
_____
_____
_____

THINGS THAT WERE HARD OR STRESSFUL TODAY:
_____
_____
_____

KIND THINGS I DID FOR MYSELF:
_____
_____
_____

OTHER THOUGHTS:
_____
_____
_____
_____
_____
_____
_____

TIME:	AS I WOKE UP			AS I WENT TO SLEEP
MOOD:				
NOTES:				

RECORD

DATE ___/___/___

AN INTENTION FOR THE DAY:

SLEPT: FROM ___:___ TO ___:___   TOTAL HOURS:___
☐ GOOD DREAMS   ☐ BAD DREAMS   ☐ NO DREAMS
NOTES:

WHAT I ATE FOR:

BREAKFAST:

LUNCH:

DINNER:

SNACKS:

NUMBER OF CUPS OF WATER I DRANK: ___

EXERCISE: FROM ___:___ TO ___:___
TOTAL MINUTES: ___
TYPE:

OTHER ACTIVITIES:

☐ JOURNALING
☐ SOCIAL TIME
☐ MEDITATION
☐ GRATITUDE
☐ TIME OUTSIDE
☐ CREATIVE WORK
☐ SPIRITUAL PRACTICE
☐ SPA TIME
☐ THERAPY
☐ ALONE TIME
☐ BEING SILLY
☐ LEARNING SOMETHING NEW
☐ LISTENING TO MUSIC
☐ COOKING
☐ CLEANING
☐ _____

REFLECT

PHYSICALLY, I FEEL:

- [ ] ENERGIZED
- [ ] WELL-RESTED
- [ ] STRONG
- [ ] LIMBER
- [ ] RELAXED
- [ ] _____

- [ ] SLUGGISH
- [ ] TIRED
- [ ] WEAK
- [ ] SORE
- [ ] STRESSED
- [ ] _____

THINGS THAT WERE FUN OR RELAXING TODAY:

_____
_____
_____

THINGS THAT WERE HARD OR STRESSFUL TODAY:

_____
_____
_____

KIND THINGS I DID FOR MYSELF:

_____
_____
_____

OTHER THOUGHTS:

_____
_____
_____
_____
_____
_____
_____

TIME:	AS I WOKE UP			AS I WENT TO SLEEP
MOOD:				
NOTES:				

RECORD

DATE ___/___/___

AN INTENTION FOR THE DAY:

SLEPT: FROM ___:___ TO ___:___   TOTAL HOURS:___

☐ GOOD DREAMS ☐ BAD DREAMS ☐ NO DREAMS

NOTES:

WHAT I ATE FOR:

BREAKFAST:

LUNCH:

DINNER:

SNACKS:

NUMBER OF CUPS OF WATER I DRANK: ___

EXERCISE: FROM ___:___ TO ___:___
TOTAL MINUTES: ___
TYPE:

OTHER ACTIVITIES:

☐ JOURNALING
☐ SOCIAL TIME
☐ MEDITATION
☐ GRATITUDE
☐ TIME OUTSIDE
☐ CREATIVE WORK

☐ SPIRITUAL PRACTICE
☐ SPA TIME
☐ THERAPY
☐ ALONE TIME
☐ BEING SILLY

☐ LEARNING SOMETHING NEW
☐ LISTENING TO MUSIC
☐ COOKING
☐ CLEANING
☐ _____

REFLECT

PHYSICALLY, I FEEL:

- [ ] ENERGIZED
- [ ] WELL-RESTED
- [ ] STRONG
- [ ] LIMBER
- [ ] RELAXED
- [ ] _____

- [ ] SLUGGISH
- [ ] TIRED
- [ ] WEAK
- [ ] SORE
- [ ] STRESSED
- [ ] _____

THINGS THAT WERE FUN OR RELAXING TODAY:
_____
_____
_____

OTHER THOUGHTS:
_____
_____
_____
_____
_____
_____
_____

THINGS THAT WERE HARD OR STRESSFUL TODAY:
_____
_____
_____

KIND THINGS I DID FOR MYSELF:
_____
_____
_____

TIME:	AS I WOKE UP			AS I WENT TO SLEEP
MOOD:				
NOTES:				

RECORD

DATE ___/___/___

AN INTENTION FOR THE DAY:

SLEPT: FROM ___:___ TO ___:___ TOTAL HOURS:___

☐ GOOD DREAMS ☐ BAD DREAMS ☐ NO DREAMS

NOTES: _____

WHAT I ATE FOR:

BREAKFAST:

LUNCH:

DINNER:

SNACKS:

NUMBER OF CUPS OF WATER I DRANK: ___

EXERCISE: FROM ___:___ TO ___:___
TOTAL MINUTES: ___
TYPE:

OTHER ACTIVITIES:

- ☐ JOURNALING
- ☐ SOCIAL TIME
- ☐ MEDITATION
- ☐ GRATITUDE
- ☐ TIME OUTSIDE
- ☐ CREATIVE WORK
- ☐ SPIRITUAL PRACTICE
- ☐ SPA TIME
- ☐ THERAPY
- ☐ ALONE TIME
- ☐ BEING SILLY
- ☐ LEARNING SOMETHING NEW
- ☐ LISTENING TO MUSIC
- ☐ COOKING
- ☐ CLEANING
- ☐ _____

REFLECT

PHYSICALLY, I FEEL:

- [ ] ENERGIZED
- [ ] WELL-RESTED
- [ ] STRONG
- [ ] LIMBER
- [ ] RELAXED
- [ ] _____

- [ ] SLUGGISH
- [ ] TIRED
- [ ] WEAK
- [ ] SORE
- [ ] STRESSED
- [ ] _____

THINGS THAT WERE FUN OR RELAXING TODAY:
_____
_____
_____

THINGS THAT WERE HARD OR STRESSFUL TODAY:
_____
_____
_____

KIND THINGS I DID FOR MYSELF:
_____
_____
_____

OTHER THOUGHTS:
_____
_____
_____
_____
_____
_____
_____
_____

TIME:	AS I WOKE UP			AS I WENT TO SLEEP
MOOD:				
NOTES:				

RECORD

DATE ___/___/___

AN INTENTION FOR THE DAY:

SLEPT: FROM ___:___ TO ___:___   TOTAL HOURS:___

☐ GOOD DREAMS   ☐ BAD DREAMS   ☐ NO DREAMS

NOTES:

WHAT I ATE FOR:

BREAKFAST:

LUNCH:

DINNER:

SNACKS:

NUMBER OF CUPS OF WATER I DRANK: ___

EXERCISE: FROM ___:___ TO ___:___
TOTAL MINUTES: ___
TYPE:

OTHER ACTIVITIES:

☐ JOURNALING
☐ SOCIAL TIME
☐ MEDITATION
☐ GRATITUDE
☐ TIME OUTSIDE
☐ CREATIVE WORK

☐ SPIRITUAL PRACTICE
☐ SPA TIME
☐ THERAPY
☐ ALONE TIME
☐ BEING SILLY

☐ LEARNING SOMETHING NEW
☐ LISTENING TO MUSIC
☐ COOKING
☐ CLEANING
☐ _____

REFLECT

PHYSICALLY, I FEEL:

- ☐ ENERGIZED
- ☐ WELL-RESTED
- ☐ STRONG
- ☐ LIMBER
- ☐ RELAXED
- ☐ _____

- ☐ SLUGGISH
- ☐ TIRED
- ☐ WEAK
- ☐ SORE
- ☐ STRESSED
- ☐ _____

THINGS THAT WERE FUN OR RELAXING TODAY:
_____
_____
_____

THINGS THAT WERE HARD OR STRESSFUL TODAY:
_____
_____
_____

KIND THINGS I DID FOR MYSELF:
_____
_____
_____

OTHER THOUGHTS:
_____
_____
_____
_____
_____
_____
_____
_____

TIME:	AS I WOKE UP			AS I WENT TO SLEEP
MOOD:				
NOTES:				

RECORD

DATE ___/___/___

AN INTENTION FOR THE DAY:

SLEPT: FROM ___:___ TO ___:___   TOTAL HOURS: ___
☐ GOOD DREAMS   ☐ BAD DREAMS   ☐ NO DREAMS
NOTES:

WHAT I ATE FOR:

BREAKFAST:	LUNCH:
DINNER:	SNACKS:

NUMBER OF CUPS OF WATER I DRANK: ___

EXERCISE: FROM ___:___ TO ___:___
TOTAL MINUTES: ___
TYPE:

OTHER ACTIVITIES:

☐ JOURNALING   ☐ SPIRITUAL PRACTICE   ☐ LEARNING SOMETHING NEW
☐ SOCIAL TIME   ☐ SPA TIME   ☐ LISTENING TO MUSIC
☐ MEDITATION   ☐ THERAPY   ☐ COOKING
☐ GRATITUDE   ☐ ALONE TIME   ☐ CLEANING
☐ TIME OUTSIDE   ☐ BEING SILLY   ☐ _____
☐ CREATIVE WORK

REFLECT

PHYSICALLY, I FEEL:

- [ ] ENERGIZED
- [ ] WELL-RESTED
- [ ] STRONG
- [ ] LIMBER
- [ ] RELAXED
- [ ] _____

- [ ] SLUGGISH
- [ ] TIRED
- [ ] WEAK
- [ ] SORE
- [ ] STRESSED
- [ ] _____

THINGS THAT WERE FUN OR RELAXING TODAY:
_____
_____
_____

THINGS THAT WERE HARD OR STRESSFUL TODAY:
_____
_____
_____

KIND THINGS I DID FOR MYSELF:
_____
_____
_____

OTHER THOUGHTS:
_____
_____
_____
_____
_____
_____
_____

TIME:	AS I WOKE UP			AS I WENT TO SLEEP
MOOD:				
NOTES:				

RECORD

DATE ___/___/___

AN INTENTION FOR THE DAY:

SLEPT: FROM ___:___ TO ___:___   TOTAL HOURS:___

☐ GOOD DREAMS   ☐ BAD DREAMS   ☐ NO DREAMS

NOTES:

WHAT I ATE FOR:

BREAKFAST:

LUNCH:

DINNER:

SNACKS:

NUMBER OF CUPS OF WATER I DRANK: ___

EXERCISE: FROM ___:___ TO ___:___
TOTAL MINUTES: ___
TYPE:

OTHER ACTIVITIES:

☐ JOURNALING
☐ SOCIAL TIME
☐ MEDITATION
☐ GRATITUDE
☐ TIME OUTSIDE
☐ CREATIVE WORK

☐ SPIRITUAL PRACTICE
☐ SPA TIME
☐ THERAPY
☐ ALONE TIME
☐ BEING SILLY

☐ LEARNING SOMETHING NEW
☐ LISTENING TO MUSIC
☐ COOKING
☐ CLEANING
☐ _____

REFLECT

PHYSICALLY, I FEEL:

- [ ] ENERGIZED
- [ ] WELL-RESTED
- [ ] STRONG
- [ ] LIMBER
- [ ] RELAXED
- [ ] _____

- [ ] SLUGGISH
- [ ] TIRED
- [ ] WEAK
- [ ] SORE
- [ ] STRESSED
- [ ] _____

THINGS THAT WERE FUN OR RELAXING TODAY:
_____
_____
_____

THINGS THAT WERE HARD OR STRESSFUL TODAY:
_____
_____
_____

KIND THINGS I DID FOR MYSELF:
_____
_____
_____

OTHER THOUGHTS:
_____
_____
_____
_____
_____
_____

TIME:	AS I WOKE UP			AS I WENT TO SLEEP
MOOD:				
NOTES:				

RECORD

DATE ___/___/___

AN INTENTION FOR THE DAY:

SLEPT: FROM ___:___ TO ___:___   TOTAL HOURS:___

☐ GOOD DREAMS   ☐ BAD DREAMS   ☐ NO DREAMS

NOTES:

WHAT I ATE FOR:

BREAKFAST:

LUNCH:

DINNER:

SNACKS:

NUMBER OF CUPS OF WATER I DRANK: ___

EXERCISE: FROM ___:___ TO ___:___
TOTAL MINUTES: ___
TYPE:

OTHER ACTIVITIES:

☐ JOURNALING
☐ SOCIAL TIME
☐ MEDITATION
☐ GRATITUDE
☐ TIME OUTSIDE
☐ CREATIVE WORK

☐ SPIRITUAL PRACTICE
☐ SPA TIME
☐ THERAPY
☐ ALONE TIME
☐ BEING SILLY

☐ LEARNING SOMETHING NEW
☐ LISTENING TO MUSIC
☐ COOKING
☐ CLEANING
☐ _____

REFLECT

PHYSICALLY, I FEEL:

- [ ] ENERGIZED
- [ ] WELL-RESTED
- [ ] STRONG
- [ ] LIMBER
- [ ] RELAXED
- [ ] _____

- [ ] SLUGGISH
- [ ] TIRED
- [ ] WEAK
- [ ] SORE
- [ ] STRESSED
- [ ] _____

THINGS THAT WERE FUN OR RELAXING TODAY:
_____
_____
_____

THINGS THAT WERE HARD OR STRESSFUL TODAY:
_____
_____
_____

KIND THINGS I DID FOR MYSELF:
_____
_____
_____

OTHER THOUGHTS:
_____
_____
_____
_____
_____
_____
_____

TIME:	AS I WOKE UP			AS I WENT TO SLEEP
MOOD:				
NOTES:				

RECORD

DATE ___/___/___

AN INTENTION FOR THE DAY:

SLEPT: FROM ___:___ TO ___:___   TOTAL HOURS:___
☐ GOOD DREAMS   ☐ BAD DREAMS   ☐ NO DREAMS
NOTES:

WHAT I ATE FOR:

BREAKFAST:

LUNCH:

DINNER:

SNACKS:

NUMBER OF CUPS OF WATER I DRANK: ___

EXERCISE: FROM ___:___ TO ___:___
TOTAL MINUTES: ___
TYPE:

OTHER ACTIVITIES:

☐ JOURNALING
☐ SOCIAL TIME
☐ MEDITATION
☐ GRATITUDE
☐ TIME OUTSIDE
☐ CREATIVE WORK

☐ SPIRITUAL PRACTICE
☐ SPA TIME
☐ THERAPY
☐ ALONE TIME
☐ BEING SILLY

☐ LEARNING SOMETHING NEW
☐ LISTENING TO MUSIC
☐ COOKING
☐ CLEANING
☐ _____

REFLECT

PHYSICALLY, I FEEL:

- [ ] ENERGIZED
- [ ] WELL-RESTED
- [ ] STRONG
- [ ] LIMBER
- [ ] RELAXED
- [ ] _____

- [ ] SLUGGISH
- [ ] TIRED
- [ ] WEAK
- [ ] SORE
- [ ] STRESSED
- [ ] _____

THINGS THAT WERE FUN OR RELAXING TODAY:
_____
_____
_____

THINGS THAT WERE HARD OR STRESSFUL TODAY:
_____
_____
_____

KIND THINGS I DID FOR MYSELF:
_____
_____
_____

OTHER THOUGHTS:
_____
_____
_____
_____
_____
_____

TIME:	AS I WOKE UP			AS I WENT TO SLEEP
MOOD:				
NOTES:				

RECORD

DATE ___/___/___

AN INTENTION FOR THE DAY:

SLEPT: FROM ___:___ TO ___:___ TOTAL HOURS:___
☐ GOOD DREAMS   ☐ BAD DREAMS   ☐ NO DREAMS
NOTES:

WHAT I ATE FOR:

BREAKFAST:

LUNCH:

DINNER:

SNACKS:

NUMBER OF CUPS OF WATER I DRANK: ___

EXERCISE: FROM ___:___ TO ___:___
TOTAL MINUTES: ___
TYPE:

OTHER ACTIVITIES:

☐ JOURNALING
☐ SOCIAL TIME
☐ MEDITATION
☐ GRATITUDE
☐ TIME OUTSIDE
☐ CREATIVE WORK

☐ SPIRITUAL PRACTICE
☐ SPA TIME
☐ THERAPY
☐ ALONE TIME
☐ BEING SILLY

☐ LEARNING SOMETHING NEW
☐ LISTENING TO MUSIC
☐ COOKING
☐ CLEANING
☐ _____

REFLECT

PHYSICALLY, I FEEL:

- [ ] ENERGIZED
- [ ] WELL-RESTED
- [ ] STRONG
- [ ] LIMBER
- [ ] RELAXED
- [ ] _____

- [ ] SLUGGISH
- [ ] TIRED
- [ ] WEAK
- [ ] SORE
- [ ] STRESSED
- [ ] _____

THINGS THAT WERE FUN OR RELAXING TODAY:
_____
_____
_____

THINGS THAT WERE HARD OR STRESSFUL TODAY:
_____
_____
_____

KIND THINGS I DID FOR MYSELF:
_____
_____
_____

OTHER THOUGHTS:
_____
_____
_____
_____
_____
_____
_____

TIME:	AS I WOKE UP			AS I WENT TO SLEEP
MOOD:				
NOTES:				

RECORD

DATE ___/___/___

AN INTENTION FOR THE DAY:

SLEPT: FROM ___:___ TO ___:___   TOTAL HOURS:___
☐ GOOD DREAMS   ☐ BAD DREAMS   ☐ NO DREAMS
NOTES:

WHAT I ATE FOR:

BREAKFAST:

LUNCH:

DINNER:

SNACKS:

NUMBER OF CUPS OF WATER I DRANK: ___

EXERCISE: FROM ___:___ TO ___:___
TOTAL MINUTES: ___
TYPE:

OTHER ACTIVITIES:

☐ JOURNALING
☐ SOCIAL TIME
☐ MEDITATION
☐ GRATITUDE
☐ TIME OUTSIDE
☐ CREATIVE WORK

☐ SPIRITUAL PRACTICE
☐ SPA TIME
☐ THERAPY
☐ ALONE TIME
☐ BEING SILLY

☐ LEARNING SOMETHING NEW
☐ LISTENING TO MUSIC
☐ COOKING
☐ CLEANING
☐ _____

REFLECT

PHYSICALLY, I FEEL:

- [ ] ENERGIZED
- [ ] WELL-RESTED
- [ ] STRONG
- [ ] LIMBER
- [ ] RELAXED
- [ ] _____

- [ ] SLUGGISH
- [ ] TIRED
- [ ] WEAK
- [ ] SORE
- [ ] STRESSED
- [ ] _____

THINGS THAT WERE FUN OR RELAXING TODAY:
_____
_____
_____

OTHER THOUGHTS:
_____
_____
_____
_____
_____
_____
_____

THINGS THAT WERE HARD OR STRESSFUL TODAY:
_____
_____
_____

KIND THINGS I DID FOR MYSELF:
_____
_____
_____

TIME:	AS I WOKE UP			AS I WENT TO SLEEP
MOOD:				
NOTES:				

RECORD

DATE ___/___/___

AN INTENTION FOR THE DAY:

SLEPT: FROM ___:___ TO ___:___   TOTAL HOURS:___

☐ GOOD DREAMS   ☐ BAD DREAMS   ☐ NO DREAMS

NOTES:

WHAT I ATE FOR:

BREAKFAST:

LUNCH:

DINNER:

SNACKS:

NUMBER OF CUPS OF WATER I DRANK:___

EXERCISE: FROM ___:___ TO ___:___
TOTAL MINUTES:___
TYPE:

OTHER ACTIVITIES:

☐ JOURNALING
☐ SOCIAL TIME
☐ MEDITATION
☐ GRATITUDE
☐ TIME OUTSIDE
☐ CREATIVE WORK

☐ SPIRITUAL PRACTICE
☐ SPA TIME
☐ THERAPY
☐ ALONE TIME
☐ BEING SILLY

☐ LEARNING SOMETHING NEW
☐ LISTENING TO MUSIC
☐ COOKING
☐ CLEANING
☐ _____

REFLECT

PHYSICALLY, I FEEL:

- [ ] ENERGIZED
- [ ] WELL-RESTED
- [ ] STRONG
- [ ] LIMBER
- [ ] RELAXED
- [ ] _____

- [ ] SLUGGISH
- [ ] TIRED
- [ ] WEAK
- [ ] SORE
- [ ] STRESSED
- [ ] _____

THINGS THAT WERE FUN OR RELAXING TODAY:
_____
_____
_____

THINGS THAT WERE HARD OR STRESSFUL TODAY:
_____
_____
_____

KIND THINGS I DID FOR MYSELF:
_____
_____
_____

OTHER THOUGHTS:
_____
_____
_____
_____
_____
_____
_____

TIME:	AS I WOKE UP			AS I WENT TO SLEEP
MOOD:				
NOTES:				

RECORD

DATE ___/___/___

AN INTENTION FOR THE DAY:

SLEPT: FROM ___:___ TO ___:___   TOTAL HOURS:___

☐ GOOD DREAMS   ☐ BAD DREAMS   ☐ NO DREAMS

NOTES:

WHAT I ATE FOR:

BREAKFAST:

LUNCH:

DINNER:

SNACKS:

NUMBER OF CUPS OF WATER I DRANK: ___

EXERCISE: FROM ___:___ TO ___:___
TOTAL MINUTES: ___
TYPE:

OTHER ACTIVITIES:

☐ JOURNALING   ☐ SPIRITUAL PRACTICE   ☐ LEARNING SOMETHING NEW
☐ SOCIAL TIME   ☐ SPA TIME   ☐ LISTENING TO MUSIC
☐ MEDITATION   ☐ THERAPY   ☐ COOKING
☐ GRATITUDE   ☐ ALONE TIME   ☐ CLEANING
☐ TIME OUTSIDE   ☐ BEING SILLY   ☐ _____
☐ CREATIVE WORK

REFLECT

PHYSICALLY, I FEEL:

- [ ] ENERGIZED
- [ ] WELL-RESTED
- [ ] STRONG
- [ ] LIMBER
- [ ] RELAXED
- [ ] _____

- [ ] SLUGGISH
- [ ] TIRED
- [ ] WEAK
- [ ] SORE
- [ ] STRESSED
- [ ] _____

THINGS THAT WERE FUN OR RELAXING TODAY:
_____
_____
_____

THINGS THAT WERE HARD OR STRESSFUL TODAY:
_____
_____
_____

KIND THINGS I DID FOR MYSELF:
_____
_____
_____

OTHER THOUGHTS:
_____
_____
_____
_____
_____
_____
_____
_____

TIME:	AS I WOKE UP			AS I WENT TO SLEEP
MOOD:				
NOTES:				

RECORD

DATE ___/___/___

AN INTENTION FOR THE DAY:

SLEPT: FROM ___:___ TO ___:___   TOTAL HOURS:___

☐ GOOD DREAMS   ☐ BAD DREAMS   ☐ NO DREAMS

NOTES:

WHAT I ATE FOR:

BREAKFAST:

LUNCH:

DINNER:

SNACKS:

NUMBER OF CUPS OF WATER I DRANK: ___

EXERCISE: FROM ___:___ TO ___:___
TOTAL MINUTES: ___
TYPE:

OTHER ACTIVITIES:

☐ JOURNALING
☐ SOCIAL TIME
☐ MEDITATION
☐ GRATITUDE
☐ TIME OUTSIDE
☐ CREATIVE WORK
☐ SPIRITUAL PRACTICE
☐ SPA TIME
☐ THERAPY
☐ ALONE TIME
☐ BEING SILLY
☐ LEARNING SOMETHING NEW
☐ LISTENING TO MUSIC
☐ COOKING
☐ CLEANING
☐ _____

REFLECT

PHYSICALLY, I FEEL:

- ☐ ENERGIZED
- ☐ WELL-RESTED
- ☐ STRONG
- ☐ LIMBER
- ☐ RELAXED
- ☐ _____

- ☐ SLUGGISH
- ☐ TIRED
- ☐ WEAK
- ☐ SORE
- ☐ STRESSED
- ☐ _____

THINGS THAT WERE FUN OR RELAXING TODAY:
_____
_____
_____

THINGS THAT WERE HARD OR STRESSFUL TODAY:
_____
_____
_____

KIND THINGS I DID FOR MYSELF:
_____
_____
_____

OTHER THOUGHTS:
_____
_____
_____
_____
_____
_____
_____
_____

TIME:	AS I WOKE UP			AS I WENT TO SLEEP
MOOD:				
NOTES:				

RECORD

DATE ___/___/___

AN INTENTION FOR THE DAY:

SLEPT: FROM ___:___ TO ___:___   TOTAL HOURS:___

☐ GOOD DREAMS   ☐ BAD DREAMS   ☐ NO DREAMS

NOTES:

WHAT I ATE FOR:

BREAKFAST:

LUNCH:

DINNER:

SNACKS:

NUMBER OF CUPS OF WATER I DRANK: ___

EXERCISE: FROM ___:___ TO ___:___
TOTAL MINUTES: ___
TYPE:

OTHER ACTIVITIES:

☐ JOURNALING   ☐ SPIRITUAL PRACTICE   ☐ LEARNING SOMETHING NEW
☐ SOCIAL TIME   ☐ SPA TIME   ☐ LISTENING TO MUSIC
☐ MEDITATION   ☐ THERAPY   ☐ COOKING
☐ GRATITUDE   ☐ ALONE TIME   ☐ CLEANING
☐ TIME OUTSIDE   ☐ BEING SILLY   ☐ _____
☐ CREATIVE WORK

REFLECT

PHYSICALLY, I FEEL:

- [ ] ENERGIZED
- [ ] WELL-RESTED
- [ ] STRONG
- [ ] LIMBER
- [ ] RELAXED
- [ ] _____

- [ ] SLUGGISH
- [ ] TIRED
- [ ] WEAK
- [ ] SORE
- [ ] STRESSED
- [ ] _____

THINGS THAT WERE FUN OR RELAXING TODAY:
_____
_____
_____

THINGS THAT WERE HARD OR STRESSFUL TODAY:
_____
_____
_____

KIND THINGS I DID FOR MYSELF:
_____
_____
_____

OTHER THOUGHTS:
_____
_____
_____
_____
_____
_____

TIME:	AS I WOKE UP			AS I WENT TO SLEEP
MOOD:				
NOTES:				

RECORD

DATE ___/___/___

AN INTENTION FOR THE DAY:

SLEPT: FROM ___:___ TO ___:___   TOTAL HOURS: ___

☐ GOOD DREAMS   ☐ BAD DREAMS   ☐ NO DREAMS

NOTES:

WHAT I ATE FOR:

BREAKFAST:

LUNCH:

DINNER:

SNACKS:

NUMBER OF CUPS OF WATER I DRANK: ___

EXERCISE: FROM ___:___ TO ___:___
TOTAL MINUTES: ___
TYPE:

OTHER ACTIVITIES:

☐ JOURNALING
☐ SOCIAL TIME
☐ MEDITATION
☐ GRATITUDE
☐ TIME OUTSIDE
☐ CREATIVE WORK

☐ SPIRITUAL PRACTICE
☐ SPA TIME
☐ THERAPY
☐ ALONE TIME
☐ BEING SILLY

☐ LEARNING SOMETHING NEW
☐ LISTENING TO MUSIC
☐ COOKING
☐ CLEANING
☐ _____

REFLECT

PHYSICALLY, I FEEL:

- [ ] ENERGIZED
- [ ] WELL-RESTED
- [ ] STRONG
- [ ] LIMBER
- [ ] RELAXED
- [ ] _____

- [ ] SLUGGISH
- [ ] TIRED
- [ ] WEAK
- [ ] SORE
- [ ] STRESSED
- [ ] _____

THINGS THAT WERE FUN OR RELAXING TODAY:
_____
_____
_____

THINGS THAT WERE HARD OR STRESSFUL TODAY:
_____
_____
_____

KIND THINGS I DID FOR MYSELF:
_____
_____
_____

OTHER THOUGHTS:
_____
_____
_____
_____
_____
_____

TIME:	AS I WOKE UP			AS I WENT TO SLEEP
MOOD:				
NOTES:				

RECORD

DATE ___/___/___

AN INTENTION FOR THE DAY:

SLEPT: FROM ___:___ TO ___:___   TOTAL HOURS:___
☐ GOOD DREAMS   ☐ BAD DREAMS   ☐ NO DREAMS
NOTES:

WHAT I ATE FOR:

BREAKFAST:

LUNCH:

DINNER:

SNACKS:

NUMBER OF CUPS OF WATER I DRANK: ___

EXERCISE: FROM ___:___ TO ___:___
TOTAL MINUTES: ___
TYPE:

OTHER ACTIVITIES:

- ☐ JOURNALING
- ☐ SOCIAL TIME
- ☐ MEDITATION
- ☐ GRATITUDE
- ☐ TIME OUTSIDE
- ☐ CREATIVE WORK
- ☐ SPIRITUAL PRACTICE
- ☐ SPA TIME
- ☐ THERAPY
- ☐ ALONE TIME
- ☐ BEING SILLY
- ☐ LEARNING SOMETHING NEW
- ☐ LISTENING TO MUSIC
- ☐ COOKING
- ☐ CLEANING
- ☐ _____

REFLECT

PHYSICALLY, I FEEL:

- ☐ ENERGIZED
- ☐ WELL-RESTED
- ☐ STRONG
- ☐ LIMBER
- ☐ RELAXED
- ☐ _____

- ☐ SLUGGISH
- ☐ TIRED
- ☐ WEAK
- ☐ SORE
- ☐ STRESSED
- ☐ _____

THINGS THAT WERE FUN OR RELAXING TODAY:
_____
_____
_____

THINGS THAT WERE HARD OR STRESSFUL TODAY:
_____
_____
_____

KIND THINGS I DID FOR MYSELF:
_____
_____
_____

OTHER THOUGHTS:
_____
_____
_____
_____
_____
_____
_____

TIME:	AS I WOKE UP			AS I WENT TO SLEEP
MOOD:				
NOTES:				

RECORD

DATE ___/___/___

AN INTENTION FOR THE DAY:

SLEPT: FROM ___:___ TO ___:___ TOTAL HOURS:___
☐ GOOD DREAMS ☐ BAD DREAMS ☐ NO DREAMS
NOTES:

WHAT I ATE FOR:

BREAKFAST:

LUNCH:

DINNER:

SNACKS:

NUMBER OF CUPS OF WATER I DRANK: ___

EXERCISE: FROM ___:___ TO ___:___
TOTAL MINUTES:___
TYPE:

OTHER ACTIVITIES:

☐ JOURNALING
☐ SOCIAL TIME
☐ MEDITATION
☐ GRATITUDE
☐ TIME OUTSIDE
☐ CREATIVE WORK

☐ SPIRITUAL PRACTICE
☐ SPA TIME
☐ THERAPY
☐ ALONE TIME
☐ BEING SILLY

☐ LEARNING SOMETHING NEW
☐ LISTENING TO MUSIC
☐ COOKING
☐ CLEANING
☐ _____

REFLECT

PHYSICALLY, I FEEL:

- [ ] ENERGIZED
- [ ] WELL-RESTED
- [ ] STRONG
- [ ] LIMBER
- [ ] RELAXED
- [ ] _____

- [ ] SLUGGISH
- [ ] TIRED
- [ ] WEAK
- [ ] SORE
- [ ] STRESSED
- [ ] _____

THINGS THAT WERE FUN OR RELAXING TODAY:
_____
_____
_____

THINGS THAT WERE HARD OR STRESSFUL TODAY:
_____
_____
_____

KIND THINGS I DID FOR MYSELF:
_____
_____
_____

OTHER THOUGHTS:
_____
_____
_____
_____
_____
_____
_____

TIME:	AS I WOKE UP			AS I WENT TO SLEEP
MOOD:				
NOTES:				

RECORD

DATE ___/___/___

AN INTENTION FOR THE DAY:

SLEPT: FROM ___:___ TO ___:___ TOTAL HOURS:___
☐ GOOD DREAMS ☐ BAD DREAMS ☐ NO DREAMS
NOTES:

WHAT I ATE FOR:

BREAKFAST:

LUNCH:

DINNER:

SNACKS:

NUMBER OF CUPS OF WATER I DRANK: ___

EXERCISE: FROM ___:___ TO ___:___
TOTAL MINUTES: ___
TYPE:

OTHER ACTIVITIES:

☐ JOURNALING
☐ SOCIAL TIME
☐ MEDITATION
☐ GRATITUDE
☐ TIME OUTSIDE
☐ CREATIVE WORK
☐ SPIRITUAL PRACTICE
☐ SPA TIME
☐ THERAPY
☐ ALONE TIME
☐ BEING SILLY
☐ LEARNING SOMETHING NEW
☐ LISTENING TO MUSIC
☐ COOKING
☐ CLEANING
☐ _____

REFLECT

PHYSICALLY, I FEEL:

- [ ] ENERGIZED
- [ ] WELL-RESTED
- [ ] STRONG
- [ ] LIMBER
- [ ] RELAXED
- [ ] _____

- [ ] SLUGGISH
- [ ] TIRED
- [ ] WEAK
- [ ] SORE
- [ ] STRESSED
- [ ] _____

THINGS THAT WERE FUN OR RELAXING TODAY:
_____
_____
_____

OTHER THOUGHTS:
_____
_____
_____

THINGS THAT WERE HARD OR STRESSFUL TODAY:
_____
_____
_____

_____
_____
_____

KIND THINGS I DID FOR MYSELF:
_____
_____
_____

TIME:	AS I WOKE UP			AS I WENT TO SLEEP
MOOD:				
NOTES:				

RECORD

DATE ___/___/___

AN INTENTION FOR THE DAY:

SLEPT: FROM ___:___ TO ___:___   TOTAL HOURS: ___
☐ GOOD DREAMS   ☐ BAD DREAMS   ☐ NO DREAMS
NOTES:

WHAT I ATE FOR:

BREAKFAST:

LUNCH:

DINNER:

SNACKS:

NUMBER OF CUPS OF WATER I DRANK: ___

EXERCISE: FROM ___:___ TO ___:___
TOTAL MINUTES: ___
TYPE:

OTHER ACTIVITIES:

☐ JOURNALING
☐ SOCIAL TIME
☐ MEDITATION
☐ GRATITUDE
☐ TIME OUTSIDE
☐ CREATIVE WORK

☐ SPIRITUAL PRACTICE
☐ SPA TIME
☐ THERAPY
☐ ALONE TIME
☐ BEING SILLY

☐ LEARNING SOMETHING NEW
☐ LISTENING TO MUSIC
☐ COOKING
☐ CLEANING
☐ _____

REFLECT

PHYSICALLY, I FEEL:

- [ ] ENERGIZED
- [ ] WELL-RESTED
- [ ] STRONG
- [ ] LIMBER
- [ ] RELAXED
- [ ] _____

- [ ] SLUGGISH
- [ ] TIRED
- [ ] WEAK
- [ ] SORE
- [ ] STRESSED
- [ ] _____

THINGS THAT WERE FUN OR RELAXING TODAY:
_____
_____
_____

THINGS THAT WERE HARD OR STRESSFUL TODAY:
_____
_____
_____

KIND THINGS I DID FOR MYSELF:
_____
_____
_____

OTHER THOUGHTS:
_____
_____
_____
_____
_____
_____
_____

TIME:	AS I WOKE UP			AS I WENT TO SLEEP
MOOD:				
NOTES:				

RECORD

DATE ___/___/___

AN INTENTION FOR THE DAY:

SLEPT: FROM ___:___ TO ___:___   TOTAL HOURS:___
☐ GOOD DREAMS ☐ BAD DREAMS ☐ NO DREAMS
NOTES:

WHAT I ATE FOR:

BREAKFAST:

LUNCH:

DINNER:

SNACKS:

NUMBER OF CUPS OF WATER I DRANK: ___

EXERCISE: FROM ___:___ TO ___:___
TOTAL MINUTES: ___
TYPE:

OTHER ACTIVITIES:

☐ JOURNALING   ☐ SPIRITUAL PRACTICE   ☐ LEARNING SOMETHING NEW
☐ SOCIAL TIME   ☐ SPA TIME   ☐ LISTENING TO MUSIC
☐ MEDITATION   ☐ THERAPY   ☐ COOKING
☐ GRATITUDE   ☐ ALONE TIME   ☐ CLEANING
☐ TIME OUTSIDE   ☐ BEING SILLY   ☐ _____
☐ CREATIVE WORK

REFLECT

PHYSICALLY, I FEEL:

- [ ] ENERGIZED
- [ ] WELL-RESTED
- [ ] STRONG
- [ ] LIMBER
- [ ] RELAXED
- [ ] _____

- [ ] SLUGGISH
- [ ] TIRED
- [ ] WEAK
- [ ] SORE
- [ ] STRESSED
- [ ] _____

THINGS THAT WERE FUN OR RELAXING TODAY:
_____
_____
_____

THINGS THAT WERE HARD OR STRESSFUL TODAY:
_____
_____
_____

KIND THINGS I DID FOR MYSELF:
_____
_____
_____

OTHER THOUGHTS:
_____
_____
_____
_____
_____
_____

TIME:	AS I WOKE UP			AS I WENT TO SLEEP
MOOD:				
NOTES:				

RECORD

DATE ___/___/___

AN INTENTION FOR THE DAY:

SLEPT: FROM ___:___ TO ___:___   TOTAL HOURS:___
☐ GOOD DREAMS   ☐ BAD DREAMS   ☐ NO DREAMS
NOTES:

WHAT I ATE FOR:

BREAKFAST:

LUNCH:

DINNER:

SNACKS:

NUMBER OF CUPS OF WATER I DRANK: ___

EXERCISE: FROM ___:___ TO ___:___
TOTAL MINUTES: ___
TYPE:

OTHER ACTIVITIES:

☐ JOURNALING
☐ SOCIAL TIME
☐ MEDITATION
☐ GRATITUDE
☐ TIME OUTSIDE
☐ CREATIVE WORK
☐ SPIRITUAL PRACTICE
☐ SPA TIME
☐ THERAPY
☐ ALONE TIME
☐ BEING SILLY
☐ LEARNING SOMETHING NEW
☐ LISTENING TO MUSIC
☐ COOKING
☐ CLEANING
☐ _____

REFLECT

PHYSICALLY, I FEEL:

- [ ] ENERGIZED
- [ ] WELL-RESTED
- [ ] STRONG
- [ ] LIMBER
- [ ] RELAXED
- [ ] _____

- [ ] SLUGGISH
- [ ] TIRED
- [ ] WEAK
- [ ] SORE
- [ ] STRESSED
- [ ] _____

THINGS THAT WERE FUN OR RELAXING TODAY:
_____
_____
_____

THINGS THAT WERE HARD OR STRESSFUL TODAY:
_____
_____
_____

KIND THINGS I DID FOR MYSELF:
_____
_____
_____

OTHER THOUGHTS:
_____
_____
_____
_____
_____
_____
_____
_____

TIME:	AS I WOKE UP			AS I WENT TO SLEEP
MOOD:				
NOTES:				

RECORD

DATE ___/___/___

AN INTENTION FOR THE DAY:

SLEPT: FROM ___:___ TO ___:___   TOTAL HOURS:___

☐ GOOD DREAMS   ☐ BAD DREAMS   ☐ NO DREAMS

NOTES:

WHAT I ATE FOR:

BREAKFAST:

LUNCH:

DINNER:

SNACKS:

NUMBER OF CUPS OF WATER I DRANK: ___

EXERCISE: FROM ___:___ TO ___:___
TOTAL MINUTES: ___
TYPE:

OTHER ACTIVITIES:

☐ JOURNALING
☐ SOCIAL TIME
☐ MEDITATION
☐ GRATITUDE
☐ TIME OUTSIDE
☐ CREATIVE WORK

☐ SPIRITUAL PRACTICE
☐ SPA TIME
☐ THERAPY
☐ ALONE TIME
☐ BEING SILLY

☐ LEARNING SOMETHING NEW
☐ LISTENING TO MUSIC
☐ COOKING
☐ CLEANING
☐ _____

REFLECT

PHYSICALLY, I FEEL:

- [ ] ENERGIZED
- [ ] WELL-RESTED
- [ ] STRONG
- [ ] LIMBER
- [ ] RELAXED
- [ ] _____

- [ ] SLUGGISH
- [ ] TIRED
- [ ] WEAK
- [ ] SORE
- [ ] STRESSED
- [ ] _____

THINGS THAT WERE FUN OR RELAXING TODAY:

_____
_____
_____

OTHER THOUGHTS:

_____
_____
_____
_____
_____
_____
_____

THINGS THAT WERE HARD OR STRESSFUL TODAY:

_____
_____
_____

KIND THINGS I DID FOR MYSELF:

_____
_____
_____

TIME:	AS I WOKE UP			AS I WENT TO SLEEP
MOOD:				
NOTES:				

RECORD

DATE ___/___/___

AN INTENTION FOR THE DAY:

SLEPT: FROM ___:___ TO ___:___ TOTAL HOURS:___

☐ GOOD DREAMS ☐ BAD DREAMS ☐ NO DREAMS

NOTES:

WHAT I ATE FOR:

BREAKFAST:

LUNCH:

DINNER:

SNACKS:

NUMBER OF CUPS OF WATER I DRANK: ___

EXERCISE: FROM ___:___ TO ___:___
TOTAL MINUTES: ___
TYPE:

OTHER ACTIVITIES:

☐ JOURNALING
☐ SOCIAL TIME
☐ MEDITATION
☐ GRATITUDE
☐ TIME OUTSIDE
☐ CREATIVE WORK

☐ SPIRITUAL PRACTICE
☐ SPA TIME
☐ THERAPY
☐ ALONE TIME
☐ BEING SILLY

☐ LEARNING SOMETHING NEW
☐ LISTENING TO MUSIC
☐ COOKING
☐ CLEANING
☐ _____

REFLECT

PHYSICALLY, I FEEL:

- [ ] ENERGIZED
- [ ] WELL-RESTED
- [ ] STRONG
- [ ] LIMBER
- [ ] RELAXED
- [ ] _____

- [ ] SLUGGISH
- [ ] TIRED
- [ ] WEAK
- [ ] SORE
- [ ] STRESSED
- [ ] _____

THINGS THAT WERE FUN OR RELAXING TODAY:
_____
_____
_____

THINGS THAT WERE HARD OR STRESSFUL TODAY:
_____
_____
_____

KIND THINGS I DID FOR MYSELF:
_____
_____
_____

OTHER THOUGHTS:
_____
_____
_____
_____
_____
_____
_____

TIME:	AS I WOKE UP			AS I WENT TO SLEEP
MOOD:				
NOTES:				

RECORD

DATE ___/___/___

AN INTENTION FOR THE DAY:

SLEPT: FROM ___:___ TO ___:___   TOTAL HOURS: ___

☐ GOOD DREAMS   ☐ BAD DREAMS   ☐ NO DREAMS

NOTES:

WHAT I ATE FOR:

BREAKFAST:

LUNCH:

DINNER:

SNACKS:

NUMBER OF CUPS OF WATER I DRANK: ___

EXERCISE: FROM ___:___ TO ___:___
TOTAL MINUTES: ___
TYPE:

OTHER ACTIVITIES:

☐ JOURNALING
☐ SOCIAL TIME
☐ MEDITATION
☐ GRATITUDE
☐ TIME OUTSIDE
☐ CREATIVE WORK

☐ SPIRITUAL PRACTICE
☐ SPA TIME
☐ THERAPY
☐ ALONE TIME
☐ BEING SILLY

☐ LEARNING SOMETHING NEW
☐ LISTENING TO MUSIC
☐ COOKING
☐ CLEANING
☐ _____

REFLECT

PHYSICALLY, I FEEL:

- [ ] ENERGIZED
- [ ] WELL-RESTED
- [ ] STRONG
- [ ] LIMBER
- [ ] RELAXED
- [ ] _____

- [ ] SLUGGISH
- [ ] TIRED
- [ ] WEAK
- [ ] SORE
- [ ] STRESSED
- [ ] _____

THINGS THAT WERE FUN OR RELAXING TODAY:
_____
_____
_____

THINGS THAT WERE HARD OR STRESSFUL TODAY:
_____
_____
_____

KIND THINGS I DID FOR MYSELF:
_____
_____
_____

OTHER THOUGHTS:
_____
_____
_____
_____
_____
_____
_____

TIME:	AS I WOKE UP			AS I WENT TO SLEEP
MOOD:				
NOTES:				

RECORD

DATE ___/___/___

AN INTENTION FOR THE DAY:

SLEPT: FROM ___:___ TO ___:___ TOTAL HOURS:___
☐ GOOD DREAMS ☐ BAD DREAMS ☐ NO DREAMS
NOTES:

WHAT I ATE FOR:

BREAKFAST:

LUNCH:

DINNER:

SNACKS:

NUMBER OF CUPS OF WATER I DRANK: ___

EXERCISE: FROM ___:___ TO ___:___
TOTAL MINUTES: ___
TYPE:

OTHER ACTIVITIES:

☐ JOURNALING
☐ SOCIAL TIME
☐ MEDITATION
☐ GRATITUDE
☐ TIME OUTSIDE
☐ CREATIVE WORK
☐ SPIRITUAL PRACTICE
☐ SPA TIME
☐ THERAPY
☐ ALONE TIME
☐ BEING SILLY
☐ LEARNING SOMETHING NEW
☐ LISTENING TO MUSIC
☐ COOKING
☐ CLEANING
☐ _____

REFLECT

PHYSICALLY, I FEEL:

- [ ] ENERGIZED
- [ ] WELL-RESTED
- [ ] STRONG
- [ ] LIMBER
- [ ] RELAXED
- [ ] _____

- [ ] SLUGGISH
- [ ] TIRED
- [ ] WEAK
- [ ] SORE
- [ ] STRESSED
- [ ] _____

THINGS THAT WERE FUN OR RELAXING TODAY:
_____
_____
_____

OTHER THOUGHTS:
_____
_____
_____
_____
_____
_____
_____

THINGS THAT WERE HARD OR STRESSFUL TODAY:
_____
_____
_____

KIND THINGS I DID FOR MYSELF:
_____
_____
_____

TIME:	AS I WOKE UP			AS I WENT TO SLEEP
MOOD:				
NOTES:				

RECORD

DATE ___/___/___

AN INTENTION FOR THE DAY:

SLEPT: FROM ___:___ TO ___:___ TOTAL HOURS:___

☐ GOOD DREAMS ☐ BAD DREAMS ☐ NO DREAMS

NOTES:

WHAT I ATE FOR:

BREAKFAST:

LUNCH:

DINNER:

SNACKS:

NUMBER OF CUPS OF WATER I DRANK: ___

EXERCISE: FROM ___:___ TO ___:___
TOTAL MINUTES: ___
TYPE:

OTHER ACTIVITIES:

☐ JOURNALING
☐ SOCIAL TIME
☐ MEDITATION
☐ GRATITUDE
☐ TIME OUTSIDE
☐ CREATIVE WORK

☐ SPIRITUAL PRACTICE
☐ SPA TIME
☐ THERAPY
☐ ALONE TIME
☐ BEING SILLY

☐ LEARNING SOMETHING NEW
☐ LISTENING TO MUSIC
☐ COOKING
☐ CLEANING
☐ _____

REFLECT

PHYSICALLY, I FEEL:

- [ ] ENERGIZED
- [ ] WELL-RESTED
- [ ] STRONG
- [ ] LIMBER
- [ ] RELAXED
- [ ] _____

- [ ] SLUGGISH
- [ ] TIRED
- [ ] WEAK
- [ ] SORE
- [ ] STRESSED
- [ ] _____

THINGS THAT WERE FUN OR RELAXING TODAY:
_____
_____
_____

THINGS THAT WERE HARD OR STRESSFUL TODAY:
_____
_____
_____

KIND THINGS I DID FOR MYSELF:
_____
_____
_____

OTHER THOUGHTS:
_____
_____
_____
_____
_____
_____
_____

TIME:	AS I WOKE UP			AS I WENT TO SLEEP
MOOD:				
NOTES:				

RECORD

DATE ___/___/___

AN INTENTION FOR THE DAY:

SLEPT: FROM ___:___ TO ___:___   TOTAL HOURS:___
☐ GOOD DREAMS   ☐ BAD DREAMS   ☐ NO DREAMS
NOTES:

WHAT I ATE FOR:

BREAKFAST:

LUNCH:

DINNER:

SNACKS:

NUMBER OF CUPS OF WATER I DRANK: ___

EXERCISE: FROM ___:___ TO ___:___
TOTAL MINUTES: ___
TYPE:

OTHER ACTIVITIES:

☐ JOURNALING
☐ SOCIAL TIME
☐ MEDITATION
☐ GRATITUDE
☐ TIME OUTSIDE
☐ CREATIVE WORK

☐ SPIRITUAL PRACTICE
☐ SPA TIME
☐ THERAPY
☐ ALONE TIME
☐ BEING SILLY

☐ LEARNING SOMETHING NEW
☐ LISTENING TO MUSIC
☐ COOKING
☐ CLEANING
☐ _____

REFLECT

PHYSICALLY, I FEEL:

- [ ] ENERGIZED
- [ ] WELL-RESTED
- [ ] STRONG
- [ ] LIMBER
- [ ] RELAXED
- [ ] _____

- [ ] SLUGGISH
- [ ] TIRED
- [ ] WEAK
- [ ] SORE
- [ ] STRESSED
- [ ] _____

THINGS THAT WERE FUN OR RELAXING TODAY:

_____
_____
_____

THINGS THAT WERE HARD OR STRESSFUL TODAY:

_____
_____
_____

KIND THINGS I DID FOR MYSELF:

_____
_____
_____

OTHER THOUGHTS:

_____
_____
_____
_____
_____
_____

TIME:	AS I WOKE UP			AS I WENT TO SLEEP
MOOD:				
NOTES:				

RECORD

DATE ___/___/___

AN INTENTION FOR THE DAY:

SLEPT: FROM ___:___ TO ___:___   TOTAL HOURS:___

☐ GOOD DREAMS   ☐ BAD DREAMS   ☐ NO DREAMS

NOTES:

WHAT I ATE FOR:

BREAKFAST:

LUNCH:

DINNER:

SNACKS:

NUMBER OF CUPS OF WATER I DRANK: ___

EXERCISE: FROM ___:___ TO ___:___
TOTAL MINUTES: ___
TYPE:

OTHER ACTIVITIES:

☐ JOURNALING
☐ SOCIAL TIME
☐ MEDITATION
☐ GRATITUDE
☐ TIME OUTSIDE
☐ CREATIVE WORK

☐ SPIRITUAL PRACTICE
☐ SPA TIME
☐ THERAPY
☐ ALONE TIME
☐ BEING SILLY

☐ LEARNING SOMETHING NEW
☐ LISTENING TO MUSIC
☐ COOKING
☐ CLEANING
☐ _____

REFLECT

PHYSICALLY, I FEEL:

- ☐ ENERGIZED
- ☐ WELL-RESTED
- ☐ STRONG
- ☐ LIMBER
- ☐ RELAXED
- ☐ _____

- ☐ SLUGGISH
- ☐ TIRED
- ☐ WEAK
- ☐ SORE
- ☐ STRESSED
- ☐ _____

THINGS THAT WERE FUN OR RELAXING TODAY:
_____
_____
_____

THINGS THAT WERE HARD OR STRESSFUL TODAY:
_____
_____
_____

KIND THINGS I DID FOR MYSELF:
_____
_____
_____

OTHER THOUGHTS:
_____
_____
_____
_____
_____
_____
_____

TIME:	AS I WOKE UP		AS I WENT TO SLEEP
MOOD:			
NOTES:			

RECORD

DATE ___/___/___

AN INTENTION FOR THE DAY:

SLEPT: FROM ___:___ TO ___:___   TOTAL HOURS:___

☐ GOOD DREAMS   ☐ BAD DREAMS   ☐ NO DREAMS

NOTES:

WHAT I ATE FOR:

BREAKFAST:

LUNCH:

DINNER:

SNACKS:

NUMBER OF CUPS OF WATER I DRANK: ___

EXERCISE: FROM ___:___ TO ___:___
TOTAL MINUTES:___
TYPE:

OTHER ACTIVITIES:

☐ JOURNALING
☐ SOCIAL TIME
☐ MEDITATION
☐ GRATITUDE
☐ TIME OUTSIDE
☐ CREATIVE WORK

☐ SPIRITUAL PRACTICE
☐ SPA TIME
☐ THERAPY
☐ ALONE TIME
☐ BEING SILLY

☐ LEARNING SOMETHING NEW
☐ LISTENING TO MUSIC
☐ COOKING
☐ CLEANING
☐ _____

REFLECT

PHYSICALLY, I FEEL:

- [ ] ENERGIZED
- [ ] WELL-RESTED
- [ ] STRONG
- [ ] LIMBER
- [ ] RELAXED
- [ ] _____

- [ ] SLUGGISH
- [ ] TIRED
- [ ] WEAK
- [ ] SORE
- [ ] STRESSED
- [ ] _____

THINGS THAT WERE FUN OR RELAXING TODAY:

_____
_____
_____

THINGS THAT WERE HARD OR STRESSFUL TODAY:

_____
_____
_____

KIND THINGS I DID FOR MYSELF:

_____
_____
_____

OTHER THOUGHTS:

_____
_____
_____
_____
_____
_____

TIME:	AS I WOKE UP			AS I WENT TO SLEEP
MOOD:				
NOTES:				

RECORD

DATE ___ / ___ / ___

AN INTENTION FOR THE DAY:

SLEPT: FROM ___ : ___ TO ___ : ___   TOTAL HOURS: ___

☐ GOOD DREAMS   ☐ BAD DREAMS   ☐ NO DREAMS

NOTES:

WHAT I ATE FOR:

BREAKFAST:

LUNCH:

DINNER:

SNACKS:

NUMBER OF CUPS OF WATER I DRANK: ___

EXERCISE: FROM ___ : ___ TO ___ : ___
TOTAL MINUTES: ___
TYPE:

OTHER ACTIVITIES:

☐ JOURNALING
☐ SOCIAL TIME
☐ MEDITATION
☐ GRATITUDE
☐ TIME OUTSIDE
☐ CREATIVE WORK

☐ SPIRITUAL PRACTICE
☐ SPA TIME
☐ THERAPY
☐ ALONE TIME
☐ BEING SILLY

☐ LEARNING SOMETHING NEW
☐ LISTENING TO MUSIC
☐ COOKING
☐ CLEANING
☐ _____

REFLECT

PHYSICALLY, I FEEL:

- [ ] ENERGIZED
- [ ] WELL-RESTED
- [ ] STRONG
- [ ] LIMBER
- [ ] RELAXED
- [ ] _____

- [ ] SLUGGISH
- [ ] TIRED
- [ ] WEAK
- [ ] SORE
- [ ] STRESSED
- [ ] _____

THINGS THAT WERE FUN OR RELAXING TODAY:
_____
_____
_____

THINGS THAT WERE HARD OR STRESSFUL TODAY:
_____
_____
_____

KIND THINGS I DID FOR MYSELF:
_____
_____
_____

OTHER THOUGHTS:
_____
_____
_____
_____
_____
_____

TIME:	AS I WOKE UP			AS I WENT TO SLEEP
MOOD:				
NOTES:				

RECORD

DATE ___/___/___

AN INTENTION FOR THE DAY:

SLEPT: FROM ___:___ TO ___:___   TOTAL HOURS: ___
☐ GOOD DREAMS   ☐ BAD DREAMS   ☐ NO DREAMS
NOTES:

WHAT I ATE FOR:

BREAKFAST:

LUNCH:

DINNER:

SNACKS:

NUMBER OF CUPS OF WATER I DRANK: ___

EXERCISE: FROM ___:___ TO ___:___
TOTAL MINUTES: ___
TYPE:

OTHER ACTIVITIES:

☐ JOURNALING
☐ SOCIAL TIME
☐ MEDITATION
☐ GRATITUDE
☐ TIME OUTSIDE
☐ CREATIVE WORK

☐ SPIRITUAL PRACTICE
☐ SPA TIME
☐ THERAPY
☐ ALONE TIME
☐ BEING SILLY

☐ LEARNING SOMETHING NEW
☐ LISTENING TO MUSIC
☐ COOKING
☐ CLEANING
☐ _____

REFLECT

PHYSICALLY, I FEEL:

- ☐ ENERGIZED
- ☐ WELL-RESTED
- ☐ STRONG
- ☐ LIMBER
- ☐ RELAXED
- ☐ _____

- ☐ SLUGGISH
- ☐ TIRED
- ☐ WEAK
- ☐ SORE
- ☐ STRESSED
- ☐ _____

THINGS THAT WERE FUN OR RELAXING TODAY:
_____
_____
_____

THINGS THAT WERE HARD OR STRESSFUL TODAY:
_____
_____
_____

KIND THINGS I DID FOR MYSELF:
_____
_____
_____

OTHER THOUGHTS:
_____
_____
_____
_____
_____
_____
_____

TIME:	AS I WOKE UP			AS I WENT TO SLEEP
MOOD:				
NOTES:				

RECORD

DATE ___/___/___

AN INTENTION FOR THE DAY:

SLEPT: FROM ___:___ TO ___:___   TOTAL HOURS:___
☐ GOOD DREAMS   ☐ BAD DREAMS   ☐ NO DREAMS
NOTES:

WHAT I ATE FOR:

BREAKFAST:

LUNCH:

DINNER:

SNACKS:

NUMBER OF CUPS OF WATER I DRANK: ___

EXERCISE: FROM ___:___ TO ___:___
TOTAL MINUTES: ___
TYPE:

OTHER ACTIVITIES:

☐ JOURNALING
☐ SOCIAL TIME
☐ MEDITATION
☐ GRATITUDE
☐ TIME OUTSIDE
☐ CREATIVE WORK

☐ SPIRITUAL PRACTICE
☐ SPA TIME
☐ THERAPY
☐ ALONE TIME
☐ BEING SILLY

☐ LEARNING SOMETHING NEW
☐ LISTENING TO MUSIC
☐ COOKING
☐ CLEANING
☐ _____

REFLECT

PHYSICALLY, I FEEL:

- [ ] ENERGIZED
- [ ] WELL-RESTED
- [ ] STRONG
- [ ] LIMBER
- [ ] RELAXED
- [ ] _____

- [ ] SLUGGISH
- [ ] TIRED
- [ ] WEAK
- [ ] SORE
- [ ] STRESSED
- [ ] _____

THINGS THAT WERE FUN OR RELAXING TODAY:
_____
_____
_____

THINGS THAT WERE HARD OR STRESSFUL TODAY:
_____
_____
_____

KIND THINGS I DID FOR MYSELF:
_____
_____
_____

OTHER THOUGHTS:
_____
_____
_____
_____
_____
_____
_____

TIME:	AS I WOKE UP			AS I WENT TO SLEEP
MOOD:				
NOTES:				

RECORD

DATE ___/___/___

AN INTENTION FOR THE DAY:

SLEPT: FROM ___:___ TO ___:___ TOTAL HOURS: ___
☐ GOOD DREAMS ☐ BAD DREAMS ☐ NO DREAMS
NOTES:

WHAT I ATE FOR:

BREAKFAST:

LUNCH:

DINNER:

SNACKS:

NUMBER OF CUPS OF WATER I DRANK: ___

EXERCISE: FROM ___:___ TO ___:___
TOTAL MINUTES: ___
TYPE:

OTHER ACTIVITIES:

☐ JOURNALING
☐ SOCIAL TIME
☐ MEDITATION
☐ GRATITUDE
☐ TIME OUTSIDE
☐ CREATIVE WORK

☐ SPIRITUAL PRACTICE
☐ SPA TIME
☐ THERAPY
☐ ALONE TIME
☐ BEING SILLY

☐ LEARNING SOMETHING NEW
☐ LISTENING TO MUSIC
☐ COOKING
☐ CLEANING
☐ _____

REFLECT

PHYSICALLY, I FEEL:

- [ ] ENERGIZED
- [ ] WELL-RESTED
- [ ] STRONG
- [ ] LIMBER
- [ ] RELAXED
- [ ] _____

- [ ] SLUGGISH
- [ ] TIRED
- [ ] WEAK
- [ ] SORE
- [ ] STRESSED
- [ ] _____

THINGS THAT WERE FUN OR RELAXING TODAY:
_____
_____
_____

THINGS THAT WERE HARD OR STRESSFUL TODAY:
_____
_____
_____

KIND THINGS I DID FOR MYSELF:
_____
_____
_____

OTHER THOUGHTS:
_____
_____
_____
_____
_____
_____

TIME:	AS I WOKE UP			AS I WENT TO SLEEP
MOOD:				
NOTES:				

RECORD

DATE ___/___/___

AN INTENTION FOR THE DAY:

SLEPT: FROM ___:___ TO ___:___ TOTAL HOURS:___

☐ GOOD DREAMS   ☐ BAD DREAMS   ☐ NO DREAMS

NOTES:

WHAT I ATE FOR:

BREAKFAST:

LUNCH:

DINNER:

SNACKS:

NUMBER OF CUPS OF WATER I DRANK: ___

EXERCISE: FROM ___:___ TO ___:___
TOTAL MINUTES: ___
TYPE:

OTHER ACTIVITIES:

☐ JOURNALING
☐ SOCIAL TIME
☐ MEDITATION
☐ GRATITUDE
☐ TIME OUTSIDE
☐ CREATIVE WORK

☐ SPIRITUAL PRACTICE
☐ SPA TIME
☐ THERAPY
☐ ALONE TIME
☐ BEING SILLY

☐ LEARNING SOMETHING NEW
☐ LISTENING TO MUSIC
☐ COOKING
☐ CLEANING
☐ _____

REFLECT

PHYSICALLY, I FEEL:

- ☐ ENERGIZED
- ☐ WELL-RESTED
- ☐ STRONG
- ☐ LIMBER
- ☐ RELAXED
- ☐ _____

- ☐ SLUGGISH
- ☐ TIRED
- ☐ WEAK
- ☐ SORE
- ☐ STRESSED
- ☐ _____

THINGS THAT WERE FUN OR RELAXING TODAY:
_____
_____
_____

THINGS THAT WERE HARD OR STRESSFUL TODAY:
_____
_____
_____

KIND THINGS I DID FOR MYSELF:
_____
_____
_____

OTHER THOUGHTS:
_____
_____
_____
_____
_____
_____
_____

TIME:	AS I WOKE UP			AS I WENT TO SLEEP
MOOD:				
NOTES:				

RECORD

DATE ___ / ___ / ___

AN INTENTION FOR THE DAY:

SLEPT: FROM ___:___ TO ___:___ TOTAL HOURS:___

☐ GOOD DREAMS   ☐ BAD DREAMS   ☐ NO DREAMS

NOTES:

WHAT I ATE FOR:

BREAKFAST:

LUNCH:

DINNER:

SNACKS:

NUMBER OF CUPS OF WATER I DRANK: ___

EXERCISE: FROM ___:___ TO ___:___
TOTAL MINUTES: ___
TYPE:

OTHER ACTIVITIES:

☐ JOURNALING
☐ SOCIAL TIME
☐ MEDITATION
☐ GRATITUDE
☐ TIME OUTSIDE
☐ CREATIVE WORK

☐ SPIRITUAL PRACTICE
☐ SPA TIME
☐ THERAPY
☐ ALONE TIME
☐ BEING SILLY

☐ LEARNING SOMETHING NEW
☐ LISTENING TO MUSIC
☐ COOKING
☐ CLEANING
☐ _____

REFLECT

PHYSICALLY, I FEEL:

- [ ] ENERGIZED
- [ ] WELL-RESTED
- [ ] STRONG
- [ ] LIMBER
- [ ] RELAXED
- [ ] _____

- [ ] SLUGGISH
- [ ] TIRED
- [ ] WEAK
- [ ] SORE
- [ ] STRESSED
- [ ] _____

THINGS THAT WERE FUN OR RELAXING TODAY:

_____
_____
_____

THINGS THAT WERE HARD OR STRESSFUL TODAY:

_____
_____
_____

KIND THINGS I DID FOR MYSELF:

_____
_____
_____

OTHER THOUGHTS:

_____
_____
_____
_____
_____
_____

TIME:	AS I WOKE UP			AS I WENT TO SLEEP
MOOD:				
NOTES:				

RECORD

DATE ___/___/___

AN INTENTION FOR THE DAY:

SLEPT: FROM ___:___ TO ___:___   TOTAL HOURS:___

☐ GOOD DREAMS   ☐ BAD DREAMS   ☐ NO DREAMS

NOTES:

WHAT I ATE FOR:

BREAKFAST:

LUNCH:

DINNER:

SNACKS:

NUMBER OF CUPS OF WATER I DRANK: ___

EXERCISE: FROM ___:___ TO ___:___
TOTAL MINUTES: ___
TYPE:

OTHER ACTIVITIES:

- ☐ JOURNALING
- ☐ SOCIAL TIME
- ☐ MEDITATION
- ☐ GRATITUDE
- ☐ TIME OUTSIDE
- ☐ CREATIVE WORK
- ☐ SPIRITUAL PRACTICE
- ☐ SPA TIME
- ☐ THERAPY
- ☐ ALONE TIME
- ☐ BEING SILLY
- ☐ LEARNING SOMETHING NEW
- ☐ LISTENING TO MUSIC
- ☐ COOKING
- ☐ CLEANING
- ☐ _____

REFLECT

PHYSICALLY, I FEEL:

- ☐ ENERGIZED
- ☐ WELL-RESTED
- ☐ STRONG
- ☐ LIMBER
- ☐ RELAXED
- ☐ _____

- ☐ SLUGGISH
- ☐ TIRED
- ☐ WEAK
- ☐ SORE
- ☐ STRESSED
- ☐ _____

THINGS THAT WERE FUN OR RELAXING TODAY:
_____
_____
_____

THINGS THAT WERE HARD OR STRESSFUL TODAY:
_____
_____
_____

KIND THINGS I DID FOR MYSELF:
_____
_____
_____

OTHER THOUGHTS:
_____
_____
_____
_____
_____
_____

TIME:	AS I WOKE UP			AS I WENT TO SLEEP
MOOD:				
NOTES:				

RECORD

DATE ___/___/___

AN INTENTION FOR THE DAY:

SLEPT: FROM ___:___ TO ___:___   TOTAL HOURS:___

☐ GOOD DREAMS   ☐ BAD DREAMS   ☐ NO DREAMS

NOTES:

WHAT I ATE FOR:

BREAKFAST:

LUNCH:

DINNER:

SNACKS:

NUMBER OF CUPS OF WATER I DRANK: ___

EXERCISE: FROM ___:___ TO ___:___
TOTAL MINUTES: ___
TYPE:

OTHER ACTIVITIES:

☐ JOURNALING
☐ SOCIAL TIME
☐ MEDITATION
☐ GRATITUDE
☐ TIME OUTSIDE
☐ CREATIVE WORK

☐ SPIRITUAL PRACTICE
☐ SPA TIME
☐ THERAPY
☐ ALONE TIME
☐ BEING SILLY

☐ LEARNING SOMETHING NEW
☐ LISTENING TO MUSIC
☐ COOKING
☐ CLEANING
☐ _____

REFLECT

PHYSICALLY, I FEEL:

- [ ] ENERGIZED
- [ ] WELL-RESTED
- [ ] STRONG
- [ ] LIMBER
- [ ] RELAXED
- [ ] _____

- [ ] SLUGGISH
- [ ] TIRED
- [ ] WEAK
- [ ] SORE
- [ ] STRESSED
- [ ] _____

THINGS THAT WERE FUN OR RELAXING TODAY:
_____
_____
_____

THINGS THAT WERE HARD OR STRESSFUL TODAY:
_____
_____
_____

KIND THINGS I DID FOR MYSELF:
_____
_____
_____

OTHER THOUGHTS:
_____
_____
_____
_____
_____
_____

TIME:	AS I WOKE UP			AS I WENT TO SLEEP
MOOD:				
NOTES:				

RECORD

DATE ___/___/___

AN INTENTION FOR THE DAY:

SLEPT: FROM ___:___ TO ___:___   TOTAL HOURS:___

☐ GOOD DREAMS ☐ BAD DREAMS ☐ NO DREAMS

NOTES:

WHAT I ATE FOR:

BREAKFAST:

LUNCH:

DINNER:

SNACKS:

NUMBER OF CUPS OF WATER I DRANK: ___

EXERCISE: FROM ___:___ TO ___:___
TOTAL MINUTES: ___
TYPE:

OTHER ACTIVITIES:

☐ JOURNALING
☐ SOCIAL TIME
☐ MEDITATION
☐ GRATITUDE
☐ TIME OUTSIDE
☐ CREATIVE WORK

☐ SPIRITUAL PRACTICE
☐ SPA TIME
☐ THERAPY
☐ ALONE TIME
☐ BEING SILLY

☐ LEARNING SOMETHING NEW
☐ LISTENING TO MUSIC
☐ COOKING
☐ CLEANING
☐ _____

REFLECT

PHYSICALLY, I FEEL:

- [ ] ENERGIZED
- [ ] WELL-RESTED
- [ ] STRONG
- [ ] LIMBER
- [ ] RELAXED
- [ ] _____

- [ ] SLUGGISH
- [ ] TIRED
- [ ] WEAK
- [ ] SORE
- [ ] STRESSED
- [ ] _____

THINGS THAT WERE FUN OR RELAXING TODAY:
_____
_____
_____

THINGS THAT WERE HARD OR STRESSFUL TODAY:
_____
_____
_____

KIND THINGS I DID FOR MYSELF:
_____
_____
_____

OTHER THOUGHTS:
_____
_____
_____
_____
_____
_____

TIME:	AS I WOKE UP			AS I WENT TO SLEEP
MOOD:				
NOTES:				

RECORD

DATE ___/___/___

AN INTENTION FOR THE DAY:

SLEPT: FROM ___:___ TO ___:___   TOTAL HOURS:___

☐ GOOD DREAMS   ☐ BAD DREAMS   ☐ NO DREAMS

NOTES:

WHAT I ATE FOR:

BREAKFAST:

LUNCH:

DINNER:

SNACKS:

NUMBER OF CUPS OF WATER I DRANK: ___

EXERCISE: FROM ___:___ TO ___:___
TOTAL MINUTES: ___
TYPE:

OTHER ACTIVITIES:

☐ JOURNALING
☐ SOCIAL TIME
☐ MEDITATION
☐ GRATITUDE
☐ TIME OUTSIDE
☐ CREATIVE WORK

☐ SPIRITUAL PRACTICE
☐ SPA TIME
☐ THERAPY
☐ ALONE TIME
☐ BEING SILLY

☐ LEARNING SOMETHING NEW
☐ LISTENING TO MUSIC
☐ COOKING
☐ CLEANING
☐ _____

REFLECT

PHYSICALLY, I FEEL:

- [ ] ENERGIZED
- [ ] WELL-RESTED
- [ ] STRONG
- [ ] LIMBER
- [ ] RELAXED
- [ ] _____

- [ ] SLUGGISH
- [ ] TIRED
- [ ] WEAK
- [ ] SORE
- [ ] STRESSED
- [ ] _____

THINGS THAT WERE FUN OR RELAXING TODAY:
_____
_____
_____

THINGS THAT WERE HARD OR STRESSFUL TODAY:
_____
_____
_____

KIND THINGS I DID FOR MYSELF:
_____
_____
_____

OTHER THOUGHTS:
_____
_____
_____
_____
_____
_____
_____

TIME:	AS I WOKE UP			AS I WENT TO SLEEP
MOOD:				
NOTES:				

RECORD

DATE ___/___/___

AN INTENTION FOR THE DAY:

SLEPT: FROM ___:___ TO ___:___ TOTAL HOURS: ___

☐ GOOD DREAMS ☐ BAD DREAMS ☐ NO DREAMS

NOTES:

WHAT I ATE FOR:

BREAKFAST:

LUNCH:

DINNER:

SNACKS:

NUMBER OF CUPS OF WATER I DRANK: ___

EXERCISE: FROM ___:___ TO ___:___
TOTAL MINUTES: ___
TYPE:

OTHER ACTIVITIES:

☐ JOURNALING
☐ SOCIAL TIME
☐ MEDITATION
☐ GRATITUDE
☐ TIME OUTSIDE
☐ CREATIVE WORK

☐ SPIRITUAL PRACTICE
☐ SPA TIME
☐ THERAPY
☐ ALONE TIME
☐ BEING SILLY

☐ LEARNING SOMETHING NEW
☐ LISTENING TO MUSIC
☐ COOKING
☐ CLEANING
☐ _____

REFLECT

PHYSICALLY, I FEEL:

- ☐ ENERGIZED
- ☐ WELL-RESTED
- ☐ STRONG
- ☐ LIMBER
- ☐ RELAXED
- ☐ _____

- ☐ SLUGGISH
- ☐ TIRED
- ☐ WEAK
- ☐ SORE
- ☐ STRESSED
- ☐ _____

THINGS THAT WERE FUN OR RELAXING TODAY:
_____
_____
_____

THINGS THAT WERE HARD OR STRESSFUL TODAY:
_____
_____
_____

KIND THINGS I DID FOR MYSELF:
_____
_____
_____

OTHER THOUGHTS:
_____
_____
_____
_____
_____
_____
_____

TIME:	AS I WOKE UP			AS I WENT TO SLEEP
MOOD:				
NOTES:				

RECORD

DATE ___/___/___

AN INTENTION FOR THE DAY:

SLEPT: FROM ___:___ TO ___:___   TOTAL HOURS:___
☐ GOOD DREAMS   ☐ BAD DREAMS   ☐ NO DREAMS
NOTES:

WHAT I ATE FOR:

BREAKFAST:

LUNCH:

DINNER:

SNACKS:

NUMBER OF CUPS OF WATER I DRANK: ___

EXERCISE: FROM ___:___ TO ___:___
TOTAL MINUTES:___
TYPE:

OTHER ACTIVITIES:

☐ JOURNALING
☐ SOCIAL TIME
☐ MEDITATION
☐ GRATITUDE
☐ TIME OUTSIDE
☐ CREATIVE WORK

☐ SPIRITUAL PRACTICE
☐ SPA TIME
☐ THERAPY
☐ ALONE TIME
☐ BEING SILLY

☐ LEARNING SOMETHING NEW
☐ LISTENING TO MUSIC
☐ COOKING
☐ CLEANING
☐ _____

REFLECT

PHYSICALLY, I FEEL:

- [ ] ENERGIZED
- [ ] WELL-RESTED
- [ ] STRONG
- [ ] LIMBER
- [ ] RELAXED
- [ ] _____

- [ ] SLUGGISH
- [ ] TIRED
- [ ] WEAK
- [ ] SORE
- [ ] STRESSED
- [ ] _____

THINGS THAT WERE FUN OR RELAXING TODAY:
_____
_____
_____

THINGS THAT WERE HARD OR STRESSFUL TODAY:
_____
_____
_____

KIND THINGS I DID FOR MYSELF:
_____
_____
_____

OTHER THOUGHTS:
_____
_____
_____
_____
_____
_____

TIME:	AS I WOKE UP			AS I WENT TO SLEEP
MOOD:				
NOTES:				

RECORD

DATE ___/___/___

AN INTENTION FOR THE DAY:

SLEPT: FROM ___:___ TO ___:___ TOTAL HOURS:___

☐ GOOD DREAMS ☐ BAD DREAMS ☐ NO DREAMS

NOTES:

WHAT I ATE FOR:

BREAKFAST:

LUNCH:

DINNER:

SNACKS:

NUMBER OF CUPS OF WATER I DRANK: ___

EXERCISE: FROM ___:___ TO ___:___
TOTAL MINUTES: ___
TYPE:

OTHER ACTIVITIES:

☐ JOURNALING
☐ SOCIAL TIME
☐ MEDITATION
☐ GRATITUDE
☐ TIME OUTSIDE
☐ CREATIVE WORK

☐ SPIRITUAL PRACTICE
☐ SPA TIME
☐ THERAPY
☐ ALONE TIME
☐ BEING SILLY

☐ LEARNING SOMETHING NEW
☐ LISTENING TO MUSIC
☐ COOKING
☐ CLEANING
☐ _____

REFLECT

PHYSICALLY, I FEEL:

- [ ] ENERGIZED
- [ ] WELL-RESTED
- [ ] STRONG
- [ ] LIMBER
- [ ] RELAXED
- [ ] _____

- [ ] SLUGGISH
- [ ] TIRED
- [ ] WEAK
- [ ] SORE
- [ ] STRESSED
- [ ] _____

THINGS THAT WERE FUN OR RELAXING TODAY:
_____
_____
_____

THINGS THAT WERE HARD OR STRESSFUL TODAY:
_____
_____
_____

KIND THINGS I DID FOR MYSELF:
_____
_____
_____

OTHER THOUGHTS:
_____
_____
_____
_____
_____
_____
_____
_____

TIME:	AS I WOKE UP			AS I WENT TO SLEEP
MOOD:				
NOTES:				

RECORD

DATE ___/___/___

AN INTENTION FOR THE DAY:

SLEPT: FROM ___:___ TO ___:___   TOTAL HOURS:___
☐ GOOD DREAMS   ☐ BAD DREAMS   ☐ NO DREAMS
NOTES:

WHAT I ATE FOR:

BREAKFAST:

LUNCH:

DINNER:

SNACKS:

NUMBER OF CUPS OF WATER I DRANK: ___

EXERCISE: FROM ___:___ TO ___:___
TOTAL MINUTES: ___
TYPE:

OTHER ACTIVITIES:

☐ JOURNALING
☐ SOCIAL TIME
☐ MEDITATION
☐ GRATITUDE
☐ TIME OUTSIDE
☐ CREATIVE WORK

☐ SPIRITUAL PRACTICE
☐ SPA TIME
☐ THERAPY
☐ ALONE TIME
☐ BEING SILLY

☐ LEARNING SOMETHING NEW
☐ LISTENING TO MUSIC
☐ COOKING
☐ CLEANING
☐ _____

REFLECT

PHYSICALLY, I FEEL:

- [ ] ENERGIZED
- [ ] WELL-RESTED
- [ ] STRONG
- [ ] LIMBER
- [ ] RELAXED
- [ ] _____

- [ ] SLUGGISH
- [ ] TIRED
- [ ] WEAK
- [ ] SORE
- [ ] STRESSED
- [ ] _____

THINGS THAT WERE FUN OR RELAXING TODAY:
_____
_____
_____

THINGS THAT WERE HARD OR STRESSFUL TODAY:
_____
_____
_____

KIND THINGS I DID FOR MYSELF:
_____
_____
_____

OTHER THOUGHTS:
_____
_____
_____
_____
_____
_____
_____

TIME:	AS I WOKE UP			AS I WENT TO SLEEP
MOOD:				
NOTES:				

RECORD

DATE ___/___/___

AN INTENTION FOR THE DAY:

SLEPT: FROM ___:___ TO ___:___   TOTAL HOURS:___

☐ GOOD DREAMS   ☐ BAD DREAMS   ☐ NO DREAMS

NOTES:

WHAT I ATE FOR:

BREAKFAST:	LUNCH:
DINNER:	SNACKS:

NUMBER OF CUPS OF WATER I DRANK: ___

EXERCISE: FROM ___:___ TO ___:___
TOTAL MINUTES: ___
TYPE:

OTHER ACTIVITIES:

☐ JOURNALING
☐ SOCIAL TIME
☐ MEDITATION
☐ GRATITUDE
☐ TIME OUTSIDE
☐ CREATIVE WORK

☐ SPIRITUAL PRACTICE
☐ SPA TIME
☐ THERAPY
☐ ALONE TIME
☐ BEING SILLY

☐ LEARNING SOMETHING NEW
☐ LISTENING TO MUSIC
☐ COOKING
☐ CLEANING
☐ _____

REFLECT

PHYSICALLY, I FEEL:

- [ ] ENERGIZED
- [ ] WELL-RESTED
- [ ] STRONG
- [ ] LIMBER
- [ ] RELAXED
- [ ] _____

- [ ] SLUGGISH
- [ ] TIRED
- [ ] WEAK
- [ ] SORE
- [ ] STRESSED
- [ ] _____

THINGS THAT WERE FUN OR RELAXING TODAY:
_____
_____
_____

THINGS THAT WERE HARD OR STRESSFUL TODAY:
_____
_____
_____

KIND THINGS I DID FOR MYSELF:
_____
_____
_____

OTHER THOUGHTS:
_____
_____
_____
_____
_____
_____
_____

TIME:	AS I WOKE UP			AS I WENT TO SLEEP
MOOD:				
NOTES:				

RECORD

DATE ___/___/___

AN INTENTION FOR THE DAY:

SLEPT: FROM ___:___ TO ___:___ TOTAL HOURS:___
☐ GOOD DREAMS ☐ BAD DREAMS ☐ NO DREAMS
NOTES:

WHAT I ATE FOR:

BREAKFAST:

LUNCH:

DINNER:

SNACKS:

NUMBER OF CUPS OF WATER I DRANK:___

EXERCISE: FROM ___:___ TO ___:___
TOTAL MINUTES:___
TYPE:

OTHER ACTIVITIES:

☐ JOURNALING
☐ SOCIAL TIME
☐ MEDITATION
☐ GRATITUDE
☐ TIME OUTSIDE
☐ CREATIVE WORK
☐ SPIRITUAL PRACTICE
☐ SPA TIME
☐ THERAPY
☐ ALONE TIME
☐ BEING SILLY
☐ LEARNING SOMETHING NEW
☐ LISTENING TO MUSIC
☐ COOKING
☐ CLEANING
☐ _____

REFLECT

PHYSICALLY, I FEEL:

- [ ] ENERGIZED
- [ ] WELL-RESTED
- [ ] STRONG
- [ ] LIMBER
- [ ] RELAXED
- [ ] _____

- [ ] SLUGGISH
- [ ] TIRED
- [ ] WEAK
- [ ] SORE
- [ ] STRESSED
- [ ] _____

THINGS THAT WERE FUN OR RELAXING TODAY:

_____
_____
_____

THINGS THAT WERE HARD OR STRESSFUL TODAY:

_____
_____
_____

KIND THINGS I DID FOR MYSELF:

_____
_____
_____

OTHER THOUGHTS:

_____
_____
_____
_____
_____

TIME:	AS I WOKE UP			AS I WENT TO SLEEP
MOOD:				
NOTES:				

RECORD

DATE ___/___/___

AN INTENTION FOR THE DAY:

SLEPT: FROM ___:___ TO ___:___   TOTAL HOURS:___

☐ GOOD DREAMS   ☐ BAD DREAMS   ☐ NO DREAMS

NOTES:

WHAT I ATE FOR:

BREAKFAST:

LUNCH:

DINNER:

SNACKS:

NUMBER OF CUPS OF WATER I DRANK: ___

EXERCISE: FROM ___:___ TO ___:___
TOTAL MINUTES: ___
TYPE:

OTHER ACTIVITIES:

☐ JOURNALING   ☐ SPIRITUAL PRACTICE   ☐ LEARNING SOMETHING NEW
☐ SOCIAL TIME   ☐ SPA TIME   ☐ LISTENING TO MUSIC
☐ MEDITATION   ☐ THERAPY   ☐ COOKING
☐ GRATITUDE   ☐ ALONE TIME   ☐ CLEANING
☐ TIME OUTSIDE   ☐ BEING SILLY   ☐ _____
☐ CREATIVE WORK

REFLECT

PHYSICALLY, I FEEL:

- [ ] ENERGIZED
- [ ] WELL-RESTED
- [ ] STRONG
- [ ] LIMBER
- [ ] RELAXED
- [ ] _____

- [ ] SLUGGISH
- [ ] TIRED
- [ ] WEAK
- [ ] SORE
- [ ] STRESSED
- [ ] _____

THINGS THAT WERE FUN OR RELAXING TODAY:
_____
_____
_____

OTHER THOUGHTS:
_____
_____
_____
_____
_____
_____

THINGS THAT WERE HARD OR STRESSFUL TODAY:
_____
_____
_____

KIND THINGS I DID FOR MYSELF:
_____
_____
_____

TIME:	AS I WOKE UP			AS I WENT TO SLEEP
MOOD:				
NOTES:				

RECORD

DATE ___/___/___

AN INTENTION FOR THE DAY:

SLEPT: FROM ___:___ TO ___:___   TOTAL HOURS:___
- [ ] GOOD DREAMS   - [ ] BAD DREAMS   - [ ] NO DREAMS
NOTES:

WHAT I ATE FOR:

BREAKFAST:

LUNCH:

DINNER:

SNACKS:

NUMBER OF CUPS OF WATER I DRANK: ___

EXERCISE: FROM ___:___ TO ___:___
TOTAL MINUTES: ___
TYPE:

OTHER ACTIVITIES:

- [ ] JOURNALING
- [ ] SOCIAL TIME
- [ ] MEDITATION
- [ ] GRATITUDE
- [ ] TIME OUTSIDE
- [ ] CREATIVE WORK
- [ ] SPIRITUAL PRACTICE
- [ ] SPA TIME
- [ ] THERAPY
- [ ] ALONE TIME
- [ ] BEING SILLY
- [ ] LEARNING SOMETHING NEW
- [ ] LISTENING TO MUSIC
- [ ] COOKING
- [ ] CLEANING
- [ ] _____

REFLECT

PHYSICALLY, I FEEL:

- [ ] ENERGIZED
- [ ] WELL-RESTED
- [ ] STRONG
- [ ] LIMBER
- [ ] RELAXED
- [ ] _____

- [ ] SLUGGISH
- [ ] TIRED
- [ ] WEAK
- [ ] SORE
- [ ] STRESSED
- [ ] _____

THINGS THAT WERE FUN OR RELAXING TODAY:
_____
_____
_____

THINGS THAT WERE HARD OR STRESSFUL TODAY:
_____
_____
_____

KIND THINGS I DID FOR MYSELF:
_____
_____
_____

OTHER THOUGHTS:
_____
_____
_____
_____
_____
_____
_____

TIME:	AS I WOKE UP			AS I WENT TO SLEEP
MOOD:				
NOTES:				

RECORD

DATE ___/___/___

AN INTENTION FOR THE DAY:

SLEPT: FROM ___:___ TO ___:___ TOTAL HOURS:___
☐ GOOD DREAMS ☐ BAD DREAMS ☐ NO DREAMS
NOTES:

WHAT I ATE FOR:

BREAKFAST:

LUNCH:

DINNER:

SNACKS:

NUMBER OF CUPS OF WATER I DRANK:___

EXERCISE: FROM ___:___ TO ___:___
TOTAL MINUTES:___
TYPE:

OTHER ACTIVITIES:

☐ JOURNALING
☐ SOCIAL TIME
☐ MEDITATION
☐ GRATITUDE
☐ TIME OUTSIDE
☐ CREATIVE WORK

☐ SPIRITUAL PRACTICE
☐ SPA TIME
☐ THERAPY
☐ ALONE TIME
☐ BEING SILLY

☐ LEARNING SOMETHING NEW
☐ LISTENING TO MUSIC
☐ COOKING
☐ CLEANING
☐ _____

REFLECT

PHYSICALLY, I FEEL:

- [ ] ENERGIZED
- [ ] WELL-RESTED
- [ ] STRONG
- [ ] LIMBER
- [ ] RELAXED
- [ ] _____

- [ ] SLUGGISH
- [ ] TIRED
- [ ] WEAK
- [ ] SORE
- [ ] STRESSED
- [ ] _____

THINGS THAT WERE FUN OR RELAXING TODAY:
_____
_____
_____

THINGS THAT WERE HARD OR STRESSFUL TODAY:
_____
_____
_____

KIND THINGS I DID FOR MYSELF:
_____
_____
_____

OTHER THOUGHTS:
_____
_____
_____
_____
_____
_____
_____

TIME:	AS I WOKE UP			AS I WENT TO SLEEP
MOOD:				
NOTES:				

RECORD

DATE ___/___/___

AN INTENTION FOR THE DAY:

SLEPT: FROM ___:___ TO ___:___   TOTAL HOURS:___

☐ GOOD DREAMS   ☐ BAD DREAMS   ☐ NO DREAMS

NOTES:

WHAT I ATE FOR:

BREAKFAST:

LUNCH:

DINNER:

SNACKS:

NUMBER OF CUPS OF WATER I DRANK: ___

EXERCISE: FROM ___:___ TO ___:___
TOTAL MINUTES: ___
TYPE:

OTHER ACTIVITIES:

☐ JOURNALING
☐ SOCIAL TIME
☐ MEDITATION
☐ GRATITUDE
☐ TIME OUTSIDE
☐ CREATIVE WORK

☐ SPIRITUAL PRACTICE
☐ SPA TIME
☐ THERAPY
☐ ALONE TIME
☐ BEING SILLY

☐ LEARNING SOMETHING NEW
☐ LISTENING TO MUSIC
☐ COOKING
☐ CLEANING
☐ _____

REFLECT

PHYSICALLY, I FEEL:

- [ ] ENERGIZED
- [ ] WELL-RESTED
- [ ] STRONG
- [ ] LIMBER
- [ ] RELAXED
- [ ] _____

- [ ] SLUGGISH
- [ ] TIRED
- [ ] WEAK
- [ ] SORE
- [ ] STRESSED
- [ ] _____

THINGS THAT WERE FUN OR RELAXING TODAY:
_____
_____
_____

THINGS THAT WERE HARD OR STRESSFUL TODAY:
_____
_____
_____

KIND THINGS I DID FOR MYSELF:
_____
_____
_____

OTHER THOUGHTS:
_____
_____
_____
_____
_____
_____
_____

TIME:	AS I WOKE UP			AS I WENT TO SLEEP
MOOD:				
NOTES:				

RECORD

DATE ___/___/___

AN INTENTION FOR THE DAY:

SLEPT: FROM ___:___ TO ___:___   TOTAL HOURS:___

☐ GOOD DREAMS   ☐ BAD DREAMS   ☐ NO DREAMS

NOTES: _____

WHAT I ATE FOR:

BREAKFAST:

LUNCH:

DINNER:

SNACKS:

NUMBER OF CUPS OF WATER I DRANK: ___

EXERCISE: FROM ___:___ TO ___:___
TOTAL MINUTES: ___
TYPE:

OTHER ACTIVITIES:

☐ JOURNALING
☐ SOCIAL TIME
☐ MEDITATION
☐ GRATITUDE
☐ TIME OUTSIDE
☐ CREATIVE WORK

☐ SPIRITUAL PRACTICE
☐ SPA TIME
☐ THERAPY
☐ ALONE TIME
☐ BEING SILLY

☐ LEARNING SOMETHING NEW
☐ LISTENING TO MUSIC
☐ COOKING
☐ CLEANING
☐ _____

REFLECT

PHYSICALLY, I FEEL:

- [ ] ENERGIZED
- [ ] WELL-RESTED
- [ ] STRONG
- [ ] LIMBER
- [ ] RELAXED
- [ ] _____

- [ ] SLUGGISH
- [ ] TIRED
- [ ] WEAK
- [ ] SORE
- [ ] STRESSED
- [ ] _____

THINGS THAT WERE FUN OR RELAXING TODAY:
_____
_____
_____

THINGS THAT WERE HARD OR STRESSFUL TODAY:
_____
_____
_____

KIND THINGS I DID FOR MYSELF:
_____
_____
_____

OTHER THOUGHTS:
_____
_____
_____
_____
_____
_____
_____

TIME:	AS I WOKE UP			AS I WENT TO SLEEP
MOOD:				
NOTES:				

RECORD

DATE ____/____/____

AN INTENTION FOR THE DAY:

SLEPT: FROM ____:____ TO ____:____   TOTAL HOURS:____

☐ GOOD DREAMS   ☐ BAD DREAMS   ☐ NO DREAMS

NOTES:

WHAT I ATE FOR:

BREAKFAST:

LUNCH:

DINNER:

SNACKS:

NUMBER OF CUPS OF WATER I DRANK: ____

EXERCISE: FROM ____:____ TO ____:____
TOTAL MINUTES: ____
TYPE:

OTHER ACTIVITIES:

☐ JOURNALING
☐ SOCIAL TIME
☐ MEDITATION
☐ GRATITUDE
☐ TIME OUTSIDE
☐ CREATIVE WORK

☐ SPIRITUAL PRACTICE
☐ SPA TIME
☐ THERAPY
☐ ALONE TIME
☐ BEING SILLY

☐ LEARNING SOMETHING NEW
☐ LISTENING TO MUSIC
☐ COOKING
☐ CLEANING
☐ _____

REFLECT

PHYSICALLY, I FEEL:

- [ ] ENERGIZED
- [ ] WELL-RESTED
- [ ] STRONG
- [ ] LIMBER
- [ ] RELAXED
- [ ] _____

- [ ] SLUGGISH
- [ ] TIRED
- [ ] WEAK
- [ ] SORE
- [ ] STRESSED
- [ ] _____

THINGS THAT WERE FUN OR RELAXING TODAY:
_____
_____
_____

THINGS THAT WERE HARD OR STRESSFUL TODAY:
_____
_____
_____

KIND THINGS I DID FOR MYSELF:
_____
_____
_____

OTHER THOUGHTS:
_____
_____
_____
_____
_____
_____
_____

TIME:	AS I WOKE UP			AS I WENT TO SLEEP
MOOD:				
NOTES:				

RECORD

DATE ___/___/___

AN INTENTION FOR THE DAY:

SLEPT: FROM ___:___ TO ___:___   TOTAL HOURS:___

☐ GOOD DREAMS   ☐ BAD DREAMS   ☐ NO DREAMS

NOTES:

WHAT I ATE FOR:

BREAKFAST:

LUNCH:

DINNER:

SNACKS:

NUMBER OF CUPS OF WATER I DRANK: ___

EXERCISE: FROM ___:___ TO ___:___
TOTAL MINUTES: ___
TYPE:

OTHER ACTIVITIES:

- ☐ JOURNALING
- ☐ SOCIAL TIME
- ☐ MEDITATION
- ☐ GRATITUDE
- ☐ TIME OUTSIDE
- ☐ CREATIVE WORK
- ☐ SPIRITUAL PRACTICE
- ☐ SPA TIME
- ☐ THERAPY
- ☐ ALONE TIME
- ☐ BEING SILLY
- ☐ LEARNING SOMETHING NEW
- ☐ LISTENING TO MUSIC
- ☐ COOKING
- ☐ CLEANING
- ☐ _____

REFLECT

PHYSICALLY, I FEEL:

- ☐ ENERGIZED
- ☐ WELL-RESTED
- ☐ STRONG
- ☐ LIMBER
- ☐ RELAXED
- ☐ _____

- ☐ SLUGGISH
- ☐ TIRED
- ☐ WEAK
- ☐ SORE
- ☐ STRESSED
- ☐ _____

THINGS THAT WERE FUN OR RELAXING TODAY:
_____
_____
_____

THINGS THAT WERE HARD OR STRESSFUL TODAY:
_____
_____
_____

KIND THINGS I DID FOR MYSELF:
_____
_____
_____

OTHER THOUGHTS:
_____
_____
_____
_____
_____
_____
_____
_____

TIME:	AS I WOKE UP			AS I WENT TO SLEEP
MOOD:				
NOTES:				

RECORD

DATE ___/___/___

AN INTENTION FOR THE DAY:

SLEPT: FROM ___:___ TO ___:___   TOTAL HOURS:___
☐ GOOD DREAMS   ☐ BAD DREAMS   ☐ NO DREAMS
NOTES:

WHAT I ATE FOR:

BREAKFAST:

LUNCH:

DINNER:

SNACKS:

NUMBER OF CUPS OF WATER I DRANK: ___

EXERCISE: FROM ___:___ TO ___:___
TOTAL MINUTES: ___
TYPE:

OTHER ACTIVITIES:

☐ JOURNALING
☐ SOCIAL TIME
☐ MEDITATION
☐ GRATITUDE
☐ TIME OUTSIDE
☐ CREATIVE WORK
☐ SPIRITUAL PRACTICE
☐ SPA TIME
☐ THERAPY
☐ ALONE TIME
☐ BEING SILLY
☐ LEARNING SOMETHING NEW
☐ LISTENING TO MUSIC
☐ COOKING
☐ CLEANING
☐ _____

REFLECT

PHYSICALLY, I FEEL:

- ☐ ENERGIZED
- ☐ WELL-RESTED
- ☐ STRONG
- ☐ LIMBER
- ☐ RELAXED
- ☐ _____

- ☐ SLUGGISH
- ☐ TIRED
- ☐ WEAK
- ☐ SORE
- ☐ STRESSED
- ☐ _____

THINGS THAT WERE FUN OR RELAXING TODAY:

_____
_____
_____

THINGS THAT WERE HARD OR STRESSFUL TODAY:

_____
_____
_____

KIND THINGS I DID FOR MYSELF:

_____
_____
_____

OTHER THOUGHTS:

_____
_____
_____
_____
_____
_____
_____

TIME:	AS I WOKE UP			AS I WENT TO SLEEP
MOOD:				
NOTES:				

RECORD

DATE ___/___/___

AN INTENTION FOR THE DAY:

SLEPT: FROM ___:___ TO ___:___   TOTAL HOURS:___

☐ GOOD DREAMS   ☐ BAD DREAMS   ☐ NO DREAMS

NOTES:

WHAT I ATE FOR:

BREAKFAST:

LUNCH:

DINNER:

SNACKS:

NUMBER OF CUPS OF WATER I DRANK: ___

EXERCISE: FROM ___:___ TO ___:___
TOTAL MINUTES: ___
TYPE:

OTHER ACTIVITIES:

☐ JOURNALING
☐ SOCIAL TIME
☐ MEDITATION
☐ GRATITUDE
☐ TIME OUTSIDE
☐ CREATIVE WORK

☐ SPIRITUAL PRACTICE
☐ SPA TIME
☐ THERAPY
☐ ALONE TIME
☐ BEING SILLY

☐ LEARNING SOMETHING NEW
☐ LISTENING TO MUSIC
☐ COOKING
☐ CLEANING
☐ _____

REFLECT

PHYSICALLY, I FEEL:

- [ ] ENERGIZED
- [ ] WELL-RESTED
- [ ] STRONG
- [ ] LIMBER
- [ ] RELAXED
- [ ] _____

- [ ] SLUGGISH
- [ ] TIRED
- [ ] WEAK
- [ ] SORE
- [ ] STRESSED
- [ ] _____

THINGS THAT WERE FUN OR RELAXING TODAY:
_____
_____
_____

THINGS THAT WERE HARD OR STRESSFUL TODAY:
_____
_____
_____

KIND THINGS I DID FOR MYSELF:
_____
_____
_____

OTHER THOUGHTS:
_____
_____
_____
_____
_____
_____
_____

TIME:	AS I WOKE UP			AS I WENT TO SLEEP
MOOD:				
NOTES:				

RECORD

DATE ___/___/___

AN INTENTION FOR THE DAY:

SLEPT: FROM ___:___ TO ___:___   TOTAL HOURS:___

☐ GOOD DREAMS   ☐ BAD DREAMS   ☐ NO DREAMS

NOTES:

WHAT I ATE FOR:

BREAKFAST:

LUNCH:

DINNER:

SNACKS:

NUMBER OF CUPS OF WATER I DRANK: ___

EXERCISE: FROM ___:___ TO ___:___
TOTAL MINUTES: ___
TYPE:

OTHER ACTIVITIES:

☐ JOURNALING
☐ SOCIAL TIME
☐ MEDITATION
☐ GRATITUDE
☐ TIME OUTSIDE
☐ CREATIVE WORK

☐ SPIRITUAL PRACTICE
☐ SPA TIME
☐ THERAPY
☐ ALONE TIME
☐ BEING SILLY

☐ LEARNING SOMETHING NEW
☐ LISTENING TO MUSIC
☐ COOKING
☐ CLEANING
☐ _____

REFLECT

PHYSICALLY, I FEEL:

- [ ] ENERGIZED
- [ ] WELL-RESTED
- [ ] STRONG
- [ ] LIMBER
- [ ] RELAXED
- [ ] _____

- [ ] SLUGGISH
- [ ] TIRED
- [ ] WEAK
- [ ] SORE
- [ ] STRESSED
- [ ] _____

THINGS THAT WERE FUN OR RELAXING TODAY:

_____
_____
_____

THINGS THAT WERE HARD OR STRESSFUL TODAY:

_____
_____
_____

KIND THINGS I DID FOR MYSELF:

_____
_____
_____

OTHER THOUGHTS:

_____
_____
_____
_____
_____
_____

TIME:	AS I WOKE UP			AS I WENT TO SLEEP
MOOD:				
NOTES:				

RECORD

DATE ___/___/___

AN INTENTION FOR THE DAY:

SLEPT: FROM ___:___ TO ___:___   TOTAL HOURS:___
☐ GOOD DREAMS   ☐ BAD DREAMS   ☐ NO DREAMS
NOTES:

WHAT I ATE FOR:

BREAKFAST:

LUNCH:

DINNER:

SNACKS:

NUMBER OF CUPS OF WATER I DRANK: ___

EXERCISE: FROM ___:___ TO ___:___
TOTAL MINUTES: ___
TYPE:

OTHER ACTIVITIES:

☐ JOURNALING
☐ SOCIAL TIME
☐ MEDITATION
☐ GRATITUDE
☐ TIME OUTSIDE
☐ CREATIVE WORK
☐ SPIRITUAL PRACTICE
☐ SPA TIME
☐ THERAPY
☐ ALONE TIME
☐ BEING SILLY
☐ LEARNING SOMETHING NEW
☐ LISTENING TO MUSIC
☐ COOKING
☐ CLEANING
☐ _____

REFLECT

PHYSICALLY, I FEEL:

- ☐ ENERGIZED
- ☐ WELL-RESTED
- ☐ STRONG
- ☐ LIMBER
- ☐ RELAXED
- ☐ _____

- ☐ SLUGGISH
- ☐ TIRED
- ☐ WEAK
- ☐ SORE
- ☐ STRESSED
- ☐ _____

THINGS THAT WERE FUN OR RELAXING TODAY:
_____
_____
_____

THINGS THAT WERE HARD OR STRESSFUL TODAY:
_____
_____
_____

OTHER THOUGHTS:
_____
_____
_____
_____
_____
_____
_____

KIND THINGS I DID FOR MYSELF:
_____
_____
_____

TIME:	AS I WOKE UP			AS I WENT TO SLEEP
MOOD:				
NOTES:				

RECORD

DATE ___/___/___

AN INTENTION FOR THE DAY:

SLEPT: FROM ___:___ TO ___:___ TOTAL HOURS:___

☐ GOOD DREAMS   ☐ BAD DREAMS   ☐ NO DREAMS

NOTES:

WHAT I ATE FOR:

BREAKFAST:

LUNCH:

DINNER:

SNACKS:

NUMBER OF CUPS OF WATER I DRANK: ___

EXERCISE: FROM ___:___ TO ___:___
TOTAL MINUTES: ___
TYPE:

OTHER ACTIVITIES:

☐ JOURNALING
☐ SOCIAL TIME
☐ MEDITATION
☐ GRATITUDE
☐ TIME OUTSIDE
☐ CREATIVE WORK

☐ SPIRITUAL PRACTICE
☐ SPA TIME
☐ THERAPY
☐ ALONE TIME
☐ BEING SILLY

☐ LEARNING SOMETHING NEW
☐ LISTENING TO MUSIC
☐ COOKING
☐ CLEANING
☐ _____

REFLECT

PHYSICALLY, I FEEL:

- [ ] ENERGIZED
- [ ] WELL-RESTED
- [ ] STRONG
- [ ] LIMBER
- [ ] RELAXED
- [ ] _____

- [ ] SLUGGISH
- [ ] TIRED
- [ ] WEAK
- [ ] SORE
- [ ] STRESSED
- [ ] _____

THINGS THAT WERE FUN OR RELAXING TODAY:
_____
_____
_____

THINGS THAT WERE HARD OR STRESSFUL TODAY:
_____
_____
_____

KIND THINGS I DID FOR MYSELF:
_____
_____
_____

OTHER THOUGHTS:
_____
_____
_____
_____
_____
_____
_____

TIME:	AS I WOKE UP			AS I WENT TO SLEEP
MOOD:				
NOTES:				

RECORD

DATE ___/___/___

AN INTENTION FOR THE DAY:

SLEPT: FROM ___:___ TO ___:___   TOTAL HOURS:___
☐ GOOD DREAMS ☐ BAD DREAMS ☐ NO DREAMS
NOTES:

WHAT I ATE FOR:

BREAKFAST:

LUNCH:

DINNER:

SNACKS:

NUMBER OF CUPS OF WATER I DRANK: ___

EXERCISE: FROM ___:___ TO ___:___
TOTAL MINUTES: ___
TYPE:

OTHER ACTIVITIES:

☐ JOURNALING
☐ SOCIAL TIME
☐ MEDITATION
☐ GRATITUDE
☐ TIME OUTSIDE
☐ CREATIVE WORK
☐ SPIRITUAL PRACTICE
☐ SPA TIME
☐ THERAPY
☐ ALONE TIME
☐ BEING SILLY
☐ LEARNING SOMETHING NEW
☐ LISTENING TO MUSIC
☐ COOKING
☐ CLEANING
☐ _____

REFLECT

PHYSICALLY, I FEEL:

- [ ] ENERGIZED
- [ ] WELL-RESTED
- [ ] STRONG
- [ ] LIMBER
- [ ] RELAXED
- [ ] _____

- [ ] SLUGGISH
- [ ] TIRED
- [ ] WEAK
- [ ] SORE
- [ ] STRESSED
- [ ] _____

THINGS THAT WERE FUN OR RELAXING TODAY:
_____
_____
_____

THINGS THAT WERE HARD OR STRESSFUL TODAY:
_____
_____
_____

KIND THINGS I DID FOR MYSELF:
_____
_____
_____

OTHER THOUGHTS:
_____
_____
_____
_____
_____
_____

TIME:	AS I WOKE UP			AS I WENT TO SLEEP
MOOD:				
NOTES:				

RECORD

DATE ___/___/___

AN INTENTION FOR THE DAY:

SLEPT: FROM ___:___ TO ___:___   TOTAL HOURS:___
☐ GOOD DREAMS ☐ BAD DREAMS ☐ NO DREAMS
NOTES:

WHAT I ATE FOR:

BREAKFAST:

LUNCH:

DINNER:

SNACKS:

NUMBER OF CUPS OF WATER I DRANK: ___

EXERCISE: FROM ___:___ TO ___:___
TOTAL MINUTES:___
TYPE:

OTHER ACTIVITIES:

☐ JOURNALING
☐ SOCIAL TIME
☐ MEDITATION
☐ GRATITUDE
☐ TIME OUTSIDE
☐ CREATIVE WORK

☐ SPIRITUAL PRACTICE
☐ SPA TIME
☐ THERAPY
☐ ALONE TIME
☐ BEING SILLY

☐ LEARNING SOMETHING NEW
☐ LISTENING TO MUSIC
☐ COOKING
☐ CLEANING
☐ _____

REFLECT

PHYSICALLY, I FEEL:

- [ ] ENERGIZED
- [ ] WELL-RESTED
- [ ] STRONG
- [ ] LIMBER
- [ ] RELAXED
- [ ] _____

- [ ] SLUGGISH
- [ ] TIRED
- [ ] WEAK
- [ ] SORE
- [ ] STRESSED
- [ ] _____

THINGS THAT WERE FUN OR RELAXING TODAY:
_____
_____
_____

THINGS THAT WERE HARD OR STRESSFUL TODAY:
_____
_____
_____

KIND THINGS I DID FOR MYSELF:
_____
_____
_____

OTHER THOUGHTS:
_____
_____
_____
_____
_____
_____
_____

TIME:	AS I WOKE UP			AS I WENT TO SLEEP
MOOD:				
NOTES:				

RECORD

DATE ___/___/___

AN INTENTION FOR THE DAY:

SLEPT: FROM ___:___ TO ___:___   TOTAL HOURS:___
☐ GOOD DREAMS ☐ BAD DREAMS ☐ NO DREAMS
NOTES:

WHAT I ATE FOR:

BREAKFAST:

LUNCH:

DINNER:

SNACKS:

NUMBER OF CUPS OF WATER I DRANK: ___

EXERCISE: FROM ___:___ TO ___:___
TOTAL MINUTES: ___
TYPE:

OTHER ACTIVITIES:

☐ JOURNALING
☐ SOCIAL TIME
☐ MEDITATION
☐ GRATITUDE
☐ TIME OUTSIDE
☐ CREATIVE WORK
☐ SPIRITUAL PRACTICE
☐ SPA TIME
☐ THERAPY
☐ ALONE TIME
☐ BEING SILLY
☐ LEARNING SOMETHING NEW
☐ LISTENING TO MUSIC
☐ COOKING
☐ CLEANING
☐ _____

REFLECT

PHYSICALLY, I FEEL:

- [ ] ENERGIZED
- [ ] WELL-RESTED
- [ ] STRONG
- [ ] LIMBER
- [ ] RELAXED
- [ ] _____

- [ ] SLUGGISH
- [ ] TIRED
- [ ] WEAK
- [ ] SORE
- [ ] STRESSED
- [ ] _____

THINGS THAT WERE FUN OR RELAXING TODAY:

THINGS THAT WERE HARD OR STRESSFUL TODAY:

KIND THINGS I DID FOR MYSELF:

OTHER THOUGHTS:

TIME:	AS I WOKE UP			AS I WENT TO SLEEP
MOOD:				
NOTES:				

RECORD

DATE ___/___/___

AN INTENTION FOR THE DAY:

SLEPT: FROM ___:___ TO ___:___   TOTAL HOURS:___

☐ GOOD DREAMS   ☐ BAD DREAMS   ☐ NO DREAMS

NOTES:

WHAT I ATE FOR:

BREAKFAST:

LUNCH:

DINNER:

SNACKS:

NUMBER OF CUPS OF WATER I DRANK:___

EXERCISE: FROM ___:___ TO ___:___
TOTAL MINUTES:___
TYPE:

OTHER ACTIVITIES:

☐ JOURNALING
☐ SOCIAL TIME
☐ MEDITATION
☐ GRATITUDE
☐ TIME OUTSIDE
☐ CREATIVE WORK

☐ SPIRITUAL PRACTICE
☐ SPA TIME
☐ THERAPY
☐ ALONE TIME
☐ BEING SILLY

☐ LEARNING SOMETHING NEW
☐ LISTENING TO MUSIC
☐ COOKING
☐ CLEANING
☐ _____

REFLECT

PHYSICALLY, I FEEL:

- ☐ ENERGIZED
- ☐ WELL-RESTED
- ☐ STRONG
- ☐ LIMBER
- ☐ RELAXED
- ☐ _____

- ☐ SLUGGISH
- ☐ TIRED
- ☐ WEAK
- ☐ SORE
- ☐ STRESSED
- ☐ _____

THINGS THAT WERE FUN OR RELAXING TODAY:
_____
_____
_____

THINGS THAT WERE HARD OR STRESSFUL TODAY:
_____
_____
_____

KIND THINGS I DID FOR MYSELF:
_____
_____
_____

OTHER THOUGHTS:
_____
_____
_____
_____
_____
_____
_____

TIME:	AS I WOKE UP			AS I WENT TO SLEEP
MOOD:				
NOTES:				

RECORD

DATE ___/___/___

AN INTENTION FOR THE DAY:

SLEPT: FROM ___:___ TO ___:___   TOTAL HOURS:___

☐ GOOD DREAMS   ☐ BAD DREAMS   ☐ NO DREAMS

NOTES:

WHAT I ATE FOR:

BREAKFAST:	LUNCH:
DINNER:	SNACKS:

NUMBER OF CUPS OF WATER I DRANK: ___

EXERCISE: FROM ___:___ TO ___:___
TOTAL MINUTES: ___
TYPE:

OTHER ACTIVITIES:

☐ JOURNALING
☐ SOCIAL TIME
☐ MEDITATION
☐ GRATITUDE
☐ TIME OUTSIDE
☐ CREATIVE WORK

☐ SPIRITUAL PRACTICE
☐ SPA TIME
☐ THERAPY
☐ ALONE TIME
☐ BEING SILLY

☐ LEARNING SOMETHING NEW
☐ LISTENING TO MUSIC
☐ COOKING
☐ CLEANING
☐ _____

REFLECT

PHYSICALLY, I FEEL:

- [ ] ENERGIZED
- [ ] WELL-RESTED
- [ ] STRONG
- [ ] LIMBER
- [ ] RELAXED
- [ ] _____

- [ ] SLUGGISH
- [ ] TIRED
- [ ] WEAK
- [ ] SORE
- [ ] STRESSED
- [ ] _____

THINGS THAT WERE FUN OR RELAXING TODAY:
_____
_____
_____

THINGS THAT WERE HARD OR STRESSFUL TODAY:
_____
_____
_____

KIND THINGS I DID FOR MYSELF:
_____
_____
_____

OTHER THOUGHTS:
_____
_____
_____
_____
_____
_____
_____
_____

TIME:	AS I WOKE UP			AS I WENT TO SLEEP
MOOD:				
NOTES:				

RECORD

DATE ___/___/___

AN INTENTION FOR THE DAY:

SLEPT: FROM ___:___ TO ___:___   TOTAL HOURS:___
☐ GOOD DREAMS   ☐ BAD DREAMS   ☐ NO DREAMS
NOTES:

WHAT I ATE FOR:

BREAKFAST:

LUNCH:

DINNER:

SNACKS:

NUMBER OF CUPS OF WATER I DRANK: ___

EXERCISE: FROM ___:___ TO ___:___
TOTAL MINUTES: ___
TYPE:

OTHER ACTIVITIES:

☐ JOURNALING
☐ SOCIAL TIME
☐ MEDITATION
☐ GRATITUDE
☐ TIME OUTSIDE
☐ CREATIVE WORK
☐ SPIRITUAL PRACTICE
☐ SPA TIME
☐ THERAPY
☐ ALONE TIME
☐ BEING SILLY
☐ LEARNING SOMETHING NEW
☐ LISTENING TO MUSIC
☐ COOKING
☐ CLEANING
☐ _____

REFLECT

PHYSICALLY, I FEEL:

- [ ] ENERGIZED
- [ ] WELL-RESTED
- [ ] STRONG
- [ ] LIMBER
- [ ] RELAXED
- [ ] _____

- [ ] SLUGGISH
- [ ] TIRED
- [ ] WEAK
- [ ] SORE
- [ ] STRESSED
- [ ] _____

THINGS THAT WERE FUN OR RELAXING TODAY:
_____
_____
_____

THINGS THAT WERE HARD OR STRESSFUL TODAY:
_____
_____
_____

KIND THINGS I DID FOR MYSELF:
_____
_____
_____

OTHER THOUGHTS:
_____
_____
_____
_____
_____
_____
_____

TIME:	AS I WOKE UP			AS I WENT TO SLEEP
MOOD:				
NOTES:				

RECORD

DATE ___/___/___

AN INTENTION FOR THE DAY:

SLEPT: FROM ___:___ TO ___:___   TOTAL HOURS:___
☐ GOOD DREAMS   ☐ BAD DREAMS   ☐ NO DREAMS
NOTES:

WHAT I ATE FOR:

BREAKFAST:

LUNCH:

DINNER:

SNACKS:

NUMBER OF CUPS OF WATER I DRANK: ___

EXERCISE: FROM ___:___ TO ___:___
TOTAL MINUTES: ___
TYPE:

OTHER ACTIVITIES:

☐ JOURNALING
☐ SOCIAL TIME
☐ MEDITATION
☐ GRATITUDE
☐ TIME OUTSIDE
☐ CREATIVE WORK

☐ SPIRITUAL PRACTICE
☐ SPA TIME
☐ THERAPY
☐ ALONE TIME
☐ BEING SILLY

☐ LEARNING SOMETHING NEW
☐ LISTENING TO MUSIC
☐ COOKING
☐ CLEANING
☐ _____

REFLECT

PHYSICALLY, I FEEL:

- [ ] ENERGIZED
- [ ] WELL-RESTED
- [ ] STRONG
- [ ] LIMBER
- [ ] RELAXED
- [ ] _____

- [ ] SLUGGISH
- [ ] TIRED
- [ ] WEAK
- [ ] SORE
- [ ] STRESSED
- [ ] _____

THINGS THAT WERE FUN OR RELAXING TODAY:
_____
_____
_____

THINGS THAT WERE HARD OR STRESSFUL TODAY:
_____
_____
_____

KIND THINGS I DID FOR MYSELF:
_____
_____
_____

OTHER THOUGHTS:
_____
_____
_____
_____
_____
_____

TIME:	AS I WOKE UP			AS I WENT TO SLEEP
MOOD:				
NOTES:				

RECORD

DATE ___/___/___

AN INTENTION FOR THE DAY:

SLEPT: FROM ___:___ TO ___:___   TOTAL HOURS:___
☐ GOOD DREAMS ☐ BAD DREAMS ☐ NO DREAMS
NOTES:

WHAT I ATE FOR:

BREAKFAST:

LUNCH:

DINNER:

SNACKS:

NUMBER OF CUPS OF WATER I DRANK: ___

EXERCISE: FROM ___:___ TO ___:___
TOTAL MINUTES: ___
TYPE:

OTHER ACTIVITIES:

☐ JOURNALING
☐ SOCIAL TIME
☐ MEDITATION
☐ GRATITUDE
☐ TIME OUTSIDE
☐ CREATIVE WORK

☐ SPIRITUAL PRACTICE
☐ SPA TIME
☐ THERAPY
☐ ALONE TIME
☐ BEING SILLY

☐ LEARNING SOMETHING NEW
☐ LISTENING TO MUSIC
☐ COOKING
☐ CLEANING
☐ _____

REFLECT

PHYSICALLY, I FEEL:

- [ ] ENERGIZED
- [ ] WELL-RESTED
- [ ] STRONG
- [ ] LIMBER
- [ ] RELAXED
- [ ] _____

- [ ] SLUGGISH
- [ ] TIRED
- [ ] WEAK
- [ ] SORE
- [ ] STRESSED
- [ ] _____

THINGS THAT WERE FUN OR RELAXING TODAY:
_____
_____
_____

THINGS THAT WERE HARD OR STRESSFUL TODAY:
_____
_____
_____

KIND THINGS I DID FOR MYSELF:
_____
_____
_____

OTHER THOUGHTS:
_____
_____
_____
_____
_____
_____
_____

TIME:	AS I WOKE UP			AS I WENT TO SLEEP
MOOD:				
NOTES:				

RECORD

DATE ___/___/___

AN INTENTION FOR THE DAY:

SLEPT: FROM ___:___ TO ___:___   TOTAL HOURS:___

☐ GOOD DREAMS   ☐ BAD DREAMS   ☐ NO DREAMS

NOTES:

WHAT I ATE FOR:

BREAKFAST:

LUNCH:

DINNER:

SNACKS:

NUMBER OF CUPS OF WATER I DRANK: ___

EXERCISE: FROM ___:___ TO ___:___
TOTAL MINUTES: ___
TYPE:

OTHER ACTIVITIES:

☐ JOURNALING
☐ SOCIAL TIME
☐ MEDITATION
☐ GRATITUDE
☐ TIME OUTSIDE
☐ CREATIVE WORK

☐ SPIRITUAL PRACTICE
☐ SPA TIME
☐ THERAPY
☐ ALONE TIME
☐ BEING SILLY

☐ LEARNING SOMETHING NEW
☐ LISTENING TO MUSIC
☐ COOKING
☐ CLEANING
☐ _____

REFLECT

PHYSICALLY, I FEEL:

- [ ] ENERGIZED
- [ ] WELL-RESTED
- [ ] STRONG
- [ ] LIMBER
- [ ] RELAXED
- [ ] _____

- [ ] SLUGGISH
- [ ] TIRED
- [ ] WEAK
- [ ] SORE
- [ ] STRESSED
- [ ] _____

THINGS THAT WERE FUN OR RELAXING TODAY:
_____
_____
_____

THINGS THAT WERE HARD OR STRESSFUL TODAY:
_____
_____
_____

KIND THINGS I DID FOR MYSELF:
_____
_____
_____

OTHER THOUGHTS:
_____
_____
_____
_____
_____
_____
_____

TIME:	AS I WOKE UP			AS I WENT TO SLEEP
MOOD:				
NOTES:				

RECORD

DATE ___/___/___

AN INTENTION FOR THE DAY:

SLEPT: FROM ___:___ TO ___:___   TOTAL HOURS:___

☐ GOOD DREAMS   ☐ BAD DREAMS   ☐ NO DREAMS

NOTES:

WHAT I ATE FOR:

BREAKFAST:

LUNCH:

DINNER:

SNACKS:

NUMBER OF CUPS OF WATER I DRANK: ___

EXERCISE: FROM ___:___ TO ___:___
TOTAL MINUTES:___
TYPE:

OTHER ACTIVITIES:

☐ JOURNALING
☐ SOCIAL TIME
☐ MEDITATION
☐ GRATITUDE
☐ TIME OUTSIDE
☐ CREATIVE WORK

☐ SPIRITUAL PRACTICE
☐ SPA TIME
☐ THERAPY
☐ ALONE TIME
☐ BEING SILLY

☐ LEARNING SOMETHING NEW
☐ LISTENING TO MUSIC
☐ COOKING
☐ CLEANING
☐ _____

REFLECT

PHYSICALLY, I FEEL:

- [ ] ENERGIZED
- [ ] WELL-RESTED
- [ ] STRONG
- [ ] LIMBER
- [ ] RELAXED
- [ ] _____

- [ ] SLUGGISH
- [ ] TIRED
- [ ] WEAK
- [ ] SORE
- [ ] STRESSED
- [ ] _____

THINGS THAT WERE FUN OR RELAXING TODAY:

_____
_____
_____

THINGS THAT WERE HARD OR STRESSFUL TODAY:

_____
_____
_____

KIND THINGS I DID FOR MYSELF:

_____
_____
_____

OTHER THOUGHTS:

_____
_____
_____
_____
_____
_____
_____

TIME:	AS I WOKE UP			AS I WENT TO SLEEP
MOOD:				
NOTES:				

RECORD

DATE ___/___/___

AN INTENTION FOR THE DAY:

SLEPT: FROM ___:___ TO ___:___   TOTAL HOURS:___
☐ GOOD DREAMS   ☐ BAD DREAMS   ☐ NO DREAMS
NOTES:

WHAT I ATE FOR:

BREAKFAST:

LUNCH:

DINNER:

SNACKS:

NUMBER OF CUPS OF WATER I DRANK: ___

EXERCISE: FROM ___:___ TO ___:___
TOTAL MINUTES: ___
TYPE:

OTHER ACTIVITIES:

☐ JOURNALING
☐ SOCIAL TIME
☐ MEDITATION
☐ GRATITUDE
☐ TIME OUTSIDE
☐ CREATIVE WORK
☐ SPIRITUAL PRACTICE
☐ SPA TIME
☐ THERAPY
☐ ALONE TIME
☐ BEING SILLY
☐ LEARNING SOMETHING NEW
☐ LISTENING TO MUSIC
☐ COOKING
☐ CLEANING
☐ _____

REFLECT

PHYSICALLY, I FEEL:

- ☐ ENERGIZED
- ☐ WELL-RESTED
- ☐ STRONG
- ☐ LIMBER
- ☐ RELAXED
- ☐ _____

- ☐ SLUGGISH
- ☐ TIRED
- ☐ WEAK
- ☐ SORE
- ☐ STRESSED
- ☐ _____

THINGS THAT WERE FUN OR RELAXING TODAY:
_____
_____
_____

THINGS THAT WERE HARD OR STRESSFUL TODAY:
_____
_____
_____

KIND THINGS I DID FOR MYSELF:
_____
_____
_____

OTHER THOUGHTS:
_____
_____
_____
_____
_____
_____

TIME:	AS I WOKE UP			AS I WENT TO SLEEP
MOOD:				
NOTES:				

RECORD

DATE ___/___/___

AN INTENTION FOR THE DAY:

SLEPT: FROM ___:___ TO ___:___   TOTAL HOURS:___

☐ GOOD DREAMS   ☐ BAD DREAMS   ☐ NO DREAMS

NOTES:

WHAT I ATE FOR:

BREAKFAST:

LUNCH:

DINNER:

SNACKS:

NUMBER OF CUPS OF WATER I DRANK: ___

EXERCISE: FROM ___:___ TO ___:___
TOTAL MINUTES: ___
TYPE:

OTHER ACTIVITIES:

☐ JOURNALING
☐ SOCIAL TIME
☐ MEDITATION
☐ GRATITUDE
☐ TIME OUTSIDE
☐ CREATIVE WORK

☐ SPIRITUAL PRACTICE
☐ SPA TIME
☐ THERAPY
☐ ALONE TIME
☐ BEING SILLY

☐ LEARNING SOMETHING NEW
☐ LISTENING TO MUSIC
☐ COOKING
☐ CLEANING
☐ _____

REFLECT

PHYSICALLY, I FEEL:

- [ ] ENERGIZED
- [ ] WELL-RESTED
- [ ] STRONG
- [ ] LIMBER
- [ ] RELAXED
- [ ] _____

- [ ] SLUGGISH
- [ ] TIRED
- [ ] WEAK
- [ ] SORE
- [ ] STRESSED
- [ ] _____

THINGS THAT WERE FUN OR RELAXING TODAY:
_____
_____
_____

THINGS THAT WERE HARD OR STRESSFUL TODAY:
_____
_____
_____

KIND THINGS I DID FOR MYSELF:
_____
_____
_____

OTHER THOUGHTS:
_____
_____
_____
_____
_____
_____
_____

TIME:	AS I WOKE UP			AS I WENT TO SLEEP
MOOD:				
NOTES:				

RECORD

DATE ___/___/___

AN INTENTION FOR THE DAY:

SLEPT: FROM ___:___ TO ___:___   TOTAL HOURS:___

☐ GOOD DREAMS   ☐ BAD DREAMS   ☐ NO DREAMS

NOTES:

WHAT I ATE FOR:

BREAKFAST:

LUNCH:

DINNER:

SNACKS:

NUMBER OF CUPS OF WATER I DRANK: ___

EXERCISE: FROM ___:___ TO ___:___
TOTAL MINUTES: ___
TYPE:

OTHER ACTIVITIES:

☐ JOURNALING
☐ SOCIAL TIME
☐ MEDITATION
☐ GRATITUDE
☐ TIME OUTSIDE
☐ CREATIVE WORK

☐ SPIRITUAL PRACTICE
☐ SPA TIME
☐ THERAPY
☐ ALONE TIME
☐ BEING SILLY

☐ LEARNING SOMETHING NEW
☐ LISTENING TO MUSIC
☐ COOKING
☐ CLEANING
☐ _____

REFLECT

PHYSICALLY, I FEEL:

- [ ] ENERGIZED
- [ ] WELL-RESTED
- [ ] STRONG
- [ ] LIMBER
- [ ] RELAXED
- [ ] _____

- [ ] SLUGGISH
- [ ] TIRED
- [ ] WEAK
- [ ] SORE
- [ ] STRESSED
- [ ] _____

THINGS THAT WERE FUN OR RELAXING TODAY:
_____
_____
_____

OTHER THOUGHTS:
_____
_____
_____
_____
_____
_____
_____

THINGS THAT WERE HARD OR STRESSFUL TODAY:
_____
_____
_____

KIND THINGS I DID FOR MYSELF:
_____
_____
_____

TIME:	AS I WOKE UP			AS I WENT TO SLEEP
MOOD:				
NOTES:				

RECORD

DATE ___/___/___

AN INTENTION FOR THE DAY:

SLEPT: FROM ___:___ TO ___:___   TOTAL HOURS:___

☐ GOOD DREAMS   ☐ BAD DREAMS   ☐ NO DREAMS

NOTES:

WHAT I ATE FOR:

BREAKFAST:

LUNCH:

DINNER:

SNACKS:

NUMBER OF CUPS OF WATER I DRANK: ___

EXERCISE: FROM ___:___ TO ___:___
TOTAL MINUTES: ___
TYPE:

OTHER ACTIVITIES:

☐ JOURNALING
☐ SOCIAL TIME
☐ MEDITATION
☐ GRATITUDE
☐ TIME OUTSIDE
☐ CREATIVE WORK

☐ SPIRITUAL PRACTICE
☐ SPA TIME
☐ THERAPY
☐ ALONE TIME
☐ BEING SILLY

☐ LEARNING SOMETHING NEW
☐ LISTENING TO MUSIC
☐ COOKING
☐ CLEANING
☐ _____

REFLECT

PHYSICALLY, I FEEL:

- [ ] ENERGIZED
- [ ] WELL-RESTED
- [ ] STRONG
- [ ] LIMBER
- [ ] RELAXED
- [ ] _____

- [ ] SLUGGISH
- [ ] TIRED
- [ ] WEAK
- [ ] SORE
- [ ] STRESSED
- [ ] _____

THINGS THAT WERE FUN OR RELAXING TODAY:
_____
_____
_____

THINGS THAT WERE HARD OR STRESSFUL TODAY:
_____
_____
_____

KIND THINGS I DID FOR MYSELF:
_____
_____
_____

OTHER THOUGHTS:
_____
_____
_____
_____
_____
_____

TIME:	AS I WOKE UP			AS I WENT TO SLEEP
MOOD:				
NOTES:				

RECORD

DATE ___/___/___

AN INTENTION FOR THE DAY:

SLEPT: FROM ___:___ TO ___:___   TOTAL HOURS:___
☐ GOOD DREAMS   ☐ BAD DREAMS   ☐ NO DREAMS
NOTES:

WHAT I ATE FOR:

BREAKFAST:	LUNCH:
DINNER:	SNACKS:

NUMBER OF CUPS OF WATER I DRANK: ___

EXERCISE: FROM ___:___ TO ___:___
TOTAL MINUTES:___
TYPE:

OTHER ACTIVITIES:

☐ JOURNALING   ☐ SPIRITUAL PRACTICE   ☐ LEARNING SOMETHING NEW
☐ SOCIAL TIME   ☐ SPA TIME   ☐ LISTENING TO MUSIC
☐ MEDITATION   ☐ THERAPY   ☐ COOKING
☐ GRATITUDE   ☐ ALONE TIME   ☐ CLEANING
☐ TIME OUTSIDE   ☐ BEING SILLY   ☐ _____
☐ CREATIVE WORK

REFLECT

PHYSICALLY, I FEEL:

- [ ] ENERGIZED
- [ ] WELL-RESTED
- [ ] STRONG
- [ ] LIMBER
- [ ] RELAXED
- [ ] _____

- [ ] SLUGGISH
- [ ] TIRED
- [ ] WEAK
- [ ] SORE
- [ ] STRESSED
- [ ] _____

THINGS THAT WERE FUN OR RELAXING TODAY:
_____
_____
_____

THINGS THAT WERE HARD OR STRESSFUL TODAY:
_____
_____
_____

KIND THINGS I DID FOR MYSELF:
_____
_____
_____

OTHER THOUGHTS:
_____
_____
_____
_____
_____
_____
_____

TIME:	AS I WOKE UP			AS I WENT TO SLEEP
MOOD:				
NOTES:				

RECORD

DATE ___/___/___

AN INTENTION FOR THE DAY:

SLEPT: FROM ___:___ TO ___:___ TOTAL HOURS:___

☐ GOOD DREAMS ☐ BAD DREAMS ☐ NO DREAMS

NOTES:

WHAT I ATE FOR:

BREAKFAST:

LUNCH:

DINNER:

SNACKS:

NUMBER OF CUPS OF WATER I DRANK: ___

EXERCISE: FROM ___:___ TO ___:___

TOTAL MINUTES: ___

TYPE:

OTHER ACTIVITIES:

☐ JOURNALING
☐ SOCIAL TIME
☐ MEDITATION
☐ GRATITUDE
☐ TIME OUTSIDE
☐ CREATIVE WORK

☐ SPIRITUAL PRACTICE
☐ SPA TIME
☐ THERAPY
☐ ALONE TIME
☐ BEING SILLY

☐ LEARNING SOMETHING NEW
☐ LISTENING TO MUSIC
☐ COOKING
☐ CLEANING
☐ _____

REFLECT

PHYSICALLY, I FEEL:

- [ ] ENERGIZED
- [ ] WELL-RESTED
- [ ] STRONG
- [ ] LIMBER
- [ ] RELAXED
- [ ] _____

- [ ] SLUGGISH
- [ ] TIRED
- [ ] WEAK
- [ ] SORE
- [ ] STRESSED
- [ ] _____

THINGS THAT WERE FUN OR RELAXING TODAY:
_____
_____
_____

THINGS THAT WERE HARD OR STRESSFUL TODAY:
_____
_____
_____

KIND THINGS I DID FOR MYSELF:
_____
_____
_____

OTHER THOUGHTS:
_____
_____
_____
_____
_____
_____

TIME:	AS I WOKE UP			AS I WENT TO SLEEP
MOOD:				
NOTES:				

RECORD

DATE ___/___/___

AN INTENTION FOR THE DAY:

SLEPT: FROM ___:___ TO ___:___   TOTAL HOURS:___
☐ GOOD DREAMS   ☐ BAD DREAMS   ☐ NO DREAMS
NOTES:

WHAT I ATE FOR:

BREAKFAST:

LUNCH:

DINNER:

SNACKS:

NUMBER OF CUPS OF WATER I DRANK: ___

EXERCISE: FROM ___:___ TO ___:___
TOTAL MINUTES: ___
TYPE:

OTHER ACTIVITIES:

☐ JOURNALING
☐ SOCIAL TIME
☐ MEDITATION
☐ GRATITUDE
☐ TIME OUTSIDE
☐ CREATIVE WORK

☐ SPIRITUAL PRACTICE
☐ SPA TIME
☐ THERAPY
☐ ALONE TIME
☐ BEING SILLY

☐ LEARNING SOMETHING NEW
☐ LISTENING TO MUSIC
☐ COOKING
☐ CLEANING
☐ _____

REFLECT

PHYSICALLY, I FEEL:

- [ ] ENERGIZED
- [ ] WELL-RESTED
- [ ] STRONG
- [ ] LIMBER
- [ ] RELAXED
- [ ] _____

- [ ] SLUGGISH
- [ ] TIRED
- [ ] WEAK
- [ ] SORE
- [ ] STRESSED
- [ ] _____

THINGS THAT WERE FUN OR RELAXING TODAY:
_____
_____
_____

OTHER THOUGHTS:
_____
_____
_____
_____
_____
_____
_____

THINGS THAT WERE HARD OR STRESSFUL TODAY:
_____
_____
_____

KIND THINGS I DID FOR MYSELF:
_____
_____
_____

TIME:	AS I WOKE UP			AS I WENT TO SLEEP
MOOD:				
NOTES:				

RECORD

DATE ___/___/___

AN INTENTION FOR THE DAY:

SLEPT: FROM ___:___ TO ___:___   TOTAL HOURS:___
☐ GOOD DREAMS   ☐ BAD DREAMS   ☐ NO DREAMS
NOTES:

WHAT I ATE FOR:

BREAKFAST:

LUNCH:

DINNER:

SNACKS:

NUMBER OF CUPS OF WATER I DRANK:___

EXERCISE: FROM ___:___ TO ___:___
TOTAL MINUTES:___
TYPE:

OTHER ACTIVITIES:

- ☐ JOURNALING
- ☐ SOCIAL TIME
- ☐ MEDITATION
- ☐ GRATITUDE
- ☐ TIME OUTSIDE
- ☐ CREATIVE WORK
- ☐ SPIRITUAL PRACTICE
- ☐ SPA TIME
- ☐ THERAPY
- ☐ ALONE TIME
- ☐ BEING SILLY
- ☐ LEARNING SOMETHING NEW
- ☐ LISTENING TO MUSIC
- ☐ COOKING
- ☐ CLEANING
- ☐ _____

REFLECT

PHYSICALLY, I FEEL:

- [ ] ENERGIZED
- [ ] WELL-RESTED
- [ ] STRONG
- [ ] LIMBER
- [ ] RELAXED
- [ ] _____

- [ ] SLUGGISH
- [ ] TIRED
- [ ] WEAK
- [ ] SORE
- [ ] STRESSED
- [ ] _____

THINGS THAT WERE FUN OR RELAXING TODAY:

OTHER THOUGHTS:

THINGS THAT WERE HARD OR STRESSFUL TODAY:

KIND THINGS I DID FOR MYSELF:

TIME:	AS I WOKE UP			AS I WENT TO SLEEP
MOOD:				
NOTES:				

RECORD

DATE ___/___/___

AN INTENTION FOR THE DAY:

SLEPT: FROM ___:___ TO ___:___   TOTAL HOURS:___

☐ GOOD DREAMS   ☐ BAD DREAMS   ☐ NO DREAMS

NOTES:

WHAT I ATE FOR:

BREAKFAST:	LUNCH:
DINNER:	SNACKS:

NUMBER OF CUPS OF WATER I DRANK: ___

EXERCISE: FROM ___:___ TO ___:___
TOTAL MINUTES:___
TYPE:

OTHER ACTIVITIES:

☐ JOURNALING   ☐ SPIRITUAL PRACTICE   ☐ LEARNING SOMETHING NEW
☐ SOCIAL TIME   ☐ SPA TIME   ☐ LISTENING TO MUSIC
☐ MEDITATION   ☐ THERAPY   ☐ COOKING
☐ GRATITUDE   ☐ ALONE TIME   ☐ CLEANING
☐ TIME OUTSIDE   ☐ BEING SILLY   ☐ _____
☐ CREATIVE WORK

REFLECT

PHYSICALLY, I FEEL:

- [ ] ENERGIZED
- [ ] WELL-RESTED
- [ ] STRONG
- [ ] LIMBER
- [ ] RELAXED
- [ ] _____

- [ ] SLUGGISH
- [ ] TIRED
- [ ] WEAK
- [ ] SORE
- [ ] STRESSED
- [ ] _____

THINGS THAT WERE FUN OR RELAXING TODAY:

_____
_____
_____

THINGS THAT WERE HARD OR STRESSFUL TODAY:

_____
_____
_____

KIND THINGS I DID FOR MYSELF:

_____
_____
_____

OTHER THOUGHTS:

_____
_____
_____
_____
_____
_____

TIME:	AS I WOKE UP			AS I WENT TO SLEEP
MOOD:				
NOTES:				

RECORD

DATE ___/___/___

AN INTENTION FOR THE DAY:

SLEPT: FROM ___:___ TO ___:___   TOTAL HOURS:___

☐ GOOD DREAMS   ☐ BAD DREAMS   ☐ NO DREAMS

NOTES:

WHAT I ATE FOR:

BREAKFAST:	LUNCH:
DINNER:	SNACKS:

NUMBER OF CUPS OF WATER I DRANK:___

EXERCISE: FROM ___:___ TO ___:___
TOTAL MINUTES:___
TYPE:

OTHER ACTIVITIES:

☐ JOURNALING   ☐ SPIRITUAL PRACTICE   ☐ LEARNING SOMETHING NEW
☐ SOCIAL TIME   ☐ SPA TIME   ☐ LISTENING TO MUSIC
☐ MEDITATION   ☐ THERAPY   ☐ COOKING
☐ GRATITUDE   ☐ ALONE TIME   ☐ CLEANING
☐ TIME OUTSIDE   ☐ BEING SILLY   ☐ _____
☐ CREATIVE WORK

REFLECT

PHYSICALLY, I FEEL:

- [ ] ENERGIZED
- [ ] WELL-RESTED
- [ ] STRONG
- [ ] LIMBER
- [ ] RELAXED
- [ ] _____

- [ ] SLUGGISH
- [ ] TIRED
- [ ] WEAK
- [ ] SORE
- [ ] STRESSED
- [ ] _____

THINGS THAT WERE FUN OR RELAXING TODAY:

_____
_____
_____

THINGS THAT WERE HARD OR STRESSFUL TODAY:

_____
_____
_____

KIND THINGS I DID FOR MYSELF:

_____
_____
_____

OTHER THOUGHTS:

_____
_____
_____
_____
_____
_____

TIME:	AS I WOKE UP			AS I WENT TO SLEEP
MOOD:				.
NOTES:				

INSIGHTS
A Mandala Journal

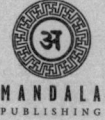

MANDALA
PUBLISHING

www.mandalaearth.com

Copyright © 2019 Mandala Publishing. All rights reserved.
This edition published by Mandala Publishing, San Rafael, California, in 2020.
Original edition first published by Mandala Publishing, San Rafael, California, in 2019.

MANUFACTURED IN CHINA
10 9 8 7 6 5 4 3 2

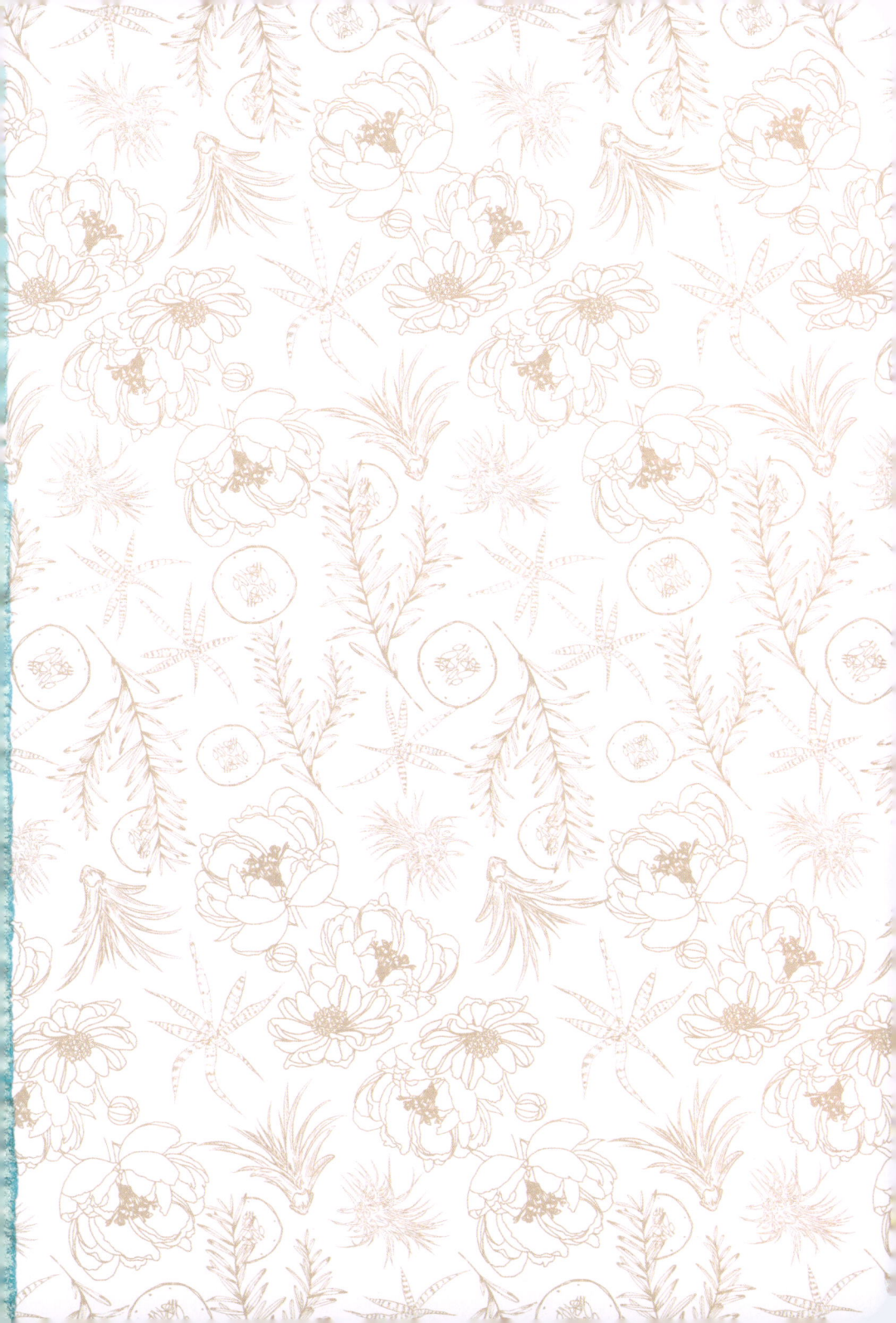